The Unmarried in
Later Life

THE UNMARRIED IN LATER LIFE

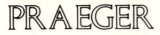Pat M. Keith

PRAEGER

New York
Westport, Connecticut
London

Library of Congress Cataloging-in-Publication Data

Keith, Pat M.
    The unmarried in later life / Pat M. Keith.
      p.   cm.
    Bibliography: p.
    Includes index.
    ISBN 0-275-92620-6 (alk. paper)
    1. Aged—United States. 2. Single people—United States.
I. Title.
  HQ1064.V5K43 1989
305.2'6—dc 19   88-28854

Library of Congress Catalog Card Number: 88-28854
ISBN: 0-275-92620-6

First published in 1989

Praeger Publishers, One Madison Avenue, New York, NY 10010
A division of Greenwood Press, Inc.

Printed in the United States of America

∞™

The paper used in this book complies with the
Permanent Paper Standard issued by the National
Information Standards Organization (Z39.48–1984).

10 9 8 7 6 5 4 3 2 1

For my "Elderlies," who have weathered transitions, to enrich my life beyond measure

Contents

Illustrations

TABLES

FIGURE

Acknowledgments

Several persons and organizations have helped in the development and preparation of this book. Some of the early analyses and writing were supported by a grant from the AARP-ANDRUS Foundation. I have also benefited from my association with and support from the College of Sciences and Humanities Research Institute, the Graduate College, and the Department of Sociology at Iowa State University.

Bud Meador, Iowa State University Statistical Laboratory, contributed valuable expertise in data management and unfailing cheerfulness. Julie Roberts typed much of the manuscript and provided many helpful suggestions. A colleague in the Department of Sociology at Iowa State University, Harry Cohen, and Mary Castles, University of Missouri–Saint Louis, and Timothy Brubaker, Miami University, shared their book-writing skills and provided unflagging encouragement.

I express my appreciation to Everett Keith for sending me my first books and to Rita Braito for the unquenchable hope that she has for us all. I give special thanks to Arthur Meyers III for his computational expertise and his endorsement and practice of feminism long before its recent renaissance.

Finally, I am ever grateful to my mother, Inez Hackler Keith, for encouraging graduate education when few women in the Ozark hills were doing so and to Roy and Mildred Ragsdale, who know how much it has meant to me.

The Unmarried in
Later Life

The Social Context of Singleness in Old Age   1

TRENDS IN SINGLENESS

This book is about being old and unmarried in the United States. It is about both men and women who were formerly married and those who have never married. But the importance of studying singleness in old age goes beyond the information on the lives of any of the individuals included in this book. More than ever before, singleness is increasingly popular. Since the 1960s, the trend has been for more adults in the United States to be single. Singleness is a recognized way of living for more people and it extends over a greater portion of the lifespan than in the past.

In popular and scientific literature singleness has been used to designate various groups of the unmarried. To some, singleness refers only to those who have never been married. To others, the definition is more encompassing. In a study of life styles, for example, the working definition of single persons used by Peter Stein (1976) included those who were not currently married or involved in an exclusive heterosexual or homosexual relationship. A legal definition of single persons and perhaps one of the least ambiguous, includes the never married, the divorced, and the widowed (Adams, 1976). Adams (1976:18) concluded that "These three groups share the common fate of not having a legal spouse and many similar practical issues of living." This book focuses on the extent to which some of the "practical issues of living" were shared as well as the ways in which they were differentiated by marital status among a sample of the unmarried in old age: the widowed, divorced/separated, and never married.

Well over one-third of the adult population of the United States is unmarried, and they are one of the most rapidly growing groups. Several demographic trends help account for the increasing numbers of the unmarried. More and more younger men and women are opting to forgo marriage at least temporarily, if not permanently. Certainly the median age at first marriage for both men and women has risen— for women from age 20.3 in 1963 to 23.3 years in 1985 and in the same period from 22.5 to 25.5 years for men (United States Bureau of the Census, 1986). This represents a dramatic increase from 28 percent of women age 20 to 24 who were single in 1960 to about 57 percent in 1984. Figures for men age 20 to 24 show smaller but nevertheless graphic increases from 53 percent who were single in 1960 to approximately 75 percent in 1984 (U.S. Bureau of the Census, 1979, 1986). It is still too early to know whether this is only a temporary decision with marriage still to come or whether there will be a lifelong commitment to singleness.

Actually, although their numbers are larger, the proportions of youth today (age 20 to 24) who have never married more closely parallel the percentages of unmarried youth at the turn of the century and a little later (United States Bureau of the Census, 1975; United States Bureau of the Census, 1981). In this sense, they share a later age at marriage with the cohort of older widowed and formerly married men and women considered in this book. The unmarried who are written about here were 20 years of age between 1925 and 1930. Early marriage was not a dominant pattern until after 1940, and age at marriage continued to decline until about 1960.

In addition to later age at marriage, another factor contributing to the increase in the unmarried in recent years is that men and women have been leaving marriages in greater numbers; for example, the proportion of persons who were divorced doubled in a recent ten year period (Norton, 1983). Although at present divorce rates are no longer increasing and have stabilized, the divorced will remain a sizable component of the unmarried population (Norton & Moorman, 1987). Thus in the population as a whole there are increasing numbers of both never married and formerly married singles. Other factors contributing to later marriage or nonmarriage include the disproportionate sex ratios in early adulthood and in middle age and beyond in some cohorts that diminish opportunities for women to marry initially and/or to remarry. And, in part, as a result of these trends, households increasingly are headed by unmarried persons, especially by women. Improved career opportunities for women and more reliable contraception may also account for later marriage or decisions to remain single.

There are some differences between men and women in patterns of singleness over the life course. Across the life cycle, for example, the total percentages of men who are unmarried do not differ a great deal until very old age when widowhood is especially prevalent (Table 1.1). By age 75, 22 percent of men are widowed. In contrast, widowhood accounts for most of the unmarried women a decade or more earlier in the 55 to 64 age group. By age 75 or over, more than three-fourths of women are unmarried. The percentage of women who have never married is fairly constant from early middle age on whereas fewer very old men have never married compared to their younger peers (Table 1.1).

Fewer older men and women are divorced than their younger counterparts. Because the proportion of younger men and women who are divorced has increased dramatically in the last decade, future cohorts of the aged will include greater proportions of the divorced (Uhlenberg & Myers, 1981). If current trends continue, when younger cohorts reach old age, as many as one-half will have experienced divorce.

There have also been significant changes within categories of the unmarried over time. In the decade between 1970 and 1980, the proportion of never-married men and women declined for three age cohorts: 45 to 54 years; 55 to 64 years; and 65 years and over (U.S. Department of Commerce, 1983). The change in the proportion of never-married men 65 years of age and over was especially graphic. In 1970, 7.5 percent of older men had never married. In the same age cohort ten years later, 4.9 percent were never married. The pattern for older never-married women was comparable as reflected in a decrease from 7.7 in 1970 to 5.9 in 1980. Reaching old age and remaining never married is becoming an increasingly rarer experience.

In contrast to the decline in the proportions of the old and never married, divorced older persons have become more commonplace. Over a 22 year period from 1960 to 1982, there were marked changes in the proportions of the divorced among both late middle-aged and older men and women (U.S. Department of Commerce, 1983). At both times more women than men were divorced although the patterns of change were comparable for both sexes. For example, in the middle years (age 45 to 64), there were 53 divorced women and 39 divorced men for each 1,000 of their married peers in 1960. In a little over two decades, there were 129 divorced women and 82 divorced men for every 1,000 married men and women in middle age. Although fewer older men and women divorced, the trends reflected in the changes over the two decades were similar. In 1960 for those age 65 years and over, 44 women and 24 men were divorced for every 1,000 married same sex peers. In contrast, at the end of a little over two decades, the number of divorced women and men had increased to 99 and 44, respectively, per 1,000 married. Whereas middle aged spouses are more likely to divorce than older couples, for both age groups there are consistent gender differences with divorce a more likely and a more sustained experience in the life course of women than of men.

These demographic changes already have had or will have an impact on the aged population in the future. Not only will the unmarried be an increasing proportion of older persons in the future (Uhlenberg & Myers, 1981), but they also will have implications for the amount and types of services needed by older persons (Beattie, 1976). Yet, except for the widowed, little is known about the unmarried in old age, especially unmarried men. With some exceptions (e.g., Braito & Anderson, 1981; Hennon, 1983; Rubinstein, 1986), research on the unmarried aged has often neglected the divorced and separated and the never married.

Even so, when all groups of the unmarried have been available for study, they often have been combined and treated as a residual category of the married. Yet, persons are unmarried in later life for diverse reasons with some statuses obviously reflecting more choice than others. Furthermore, over the life course of persons who are now old, attitudes toward the unmarried have changed somewhat.

SINGLENESS AND ADULTHOOD: HISTORICAL CONTEXT AND EVALUATIONS OF THE UNMARRIED

Although there are trends toward increases in singleness, whether formerly married or never married, the social and historical context in which the older unmarried studied here reached adulthood was characterized by negative evaluations of singleness and by the expectation that most would marry and remain married until the death of a spouse (Nimkoff, 1934).

Pressures to marry and the stigma of singleness have some of their origins in the early history of the United States in which leaders of the country hoped to increase the population as rapidly as possible. In New England, the expectation was that all would marry, marry young, and remain married. To accomplish this, singleness was actively discouraged in a number of ways. Sanctions for nonmarriage were both social and economic. Young women who were not married by age 20 were described as "stale maids" or in Puritan society, those who were unmarried when they reached their twenty-fifth birthday were said to be "antient maids" (Calhoun, 1917). Older unmarried women were targets for ridicule, viewed as failures, and frequently relegated to lives of unpaid drudgery with families of married siblings. What happened in the lives of these older women contributed to stereotypes of the unmarried in the literature of the period. They were described as sour, prim, mannish maidens, neurotic spinsters, old maids, and busybodies.

Unmarried women were not alone in being objects of ridicule and pity. There was little tolerance of the unmarried of either sex, and bachelors also were victims of harsh disapproval. Whereas some communities provided free land to induce persons to marry, in general, the alternatives to marriage were grim because those who could not offer good reasons for not marrying were regarded as little above the criminal class. Strong sanctions then were directed toward the unmarried in the form of taxation and not being permitted to live alone; in fact, certain families were licensed to provide appropriate living quarters in which the unmarried could be kept under close surveillance to insure conformity to acceptable standards of behavior (Nimkoff, 1934). In Hartford, Connecticut, for example, unmarried men were taxed 20 shillings a week, and unmarried men and women were required to live with licensed families. That the unmarried were not permitted to "diet or lodge alone" and were under strict supervision to ensure that they kept "good order day and night or otherwise" (Calhoun, 1917) gave early support to the notion that the unmarried were not to be viewed as adults. Perhaps forecasting the better economic fortunes of married than single men still prevalent today, Franklin (1745) advised that "a single man has not nearly the value he would have in that state of union." Without the help and assistance of a spouse and children on a farm or business and combined with the penalties of the bachelor tax, the single man was indeed disadvantaged like the "odd half of a pair of scissors" (Franklin, 1745).

The reasons for nonmarriage suggested in both earlier and later literature are, for the most part, derogatory and only serve to reinforce stereotypes of singleness as a deviant status. Consider, for example, some of the reasons Kuhn (1948) posited for remaining single about two centuries after Franklin:

1. hostile attitudes toward marriage or toward members of the opposite sex that may have their origins in childhood experiences;
2. homosexuality;
3. personality factors that may disqualify persons for marriage such as withdrawing from social relationships, dwelling in fantasy worlds, suspiciousness, lack of flexibility, compulsiveness;
4. emotional fixation on either parent;
5. poor health or unattractive physique;
6. ineptness in the dating process;
7. unrealistic expectations about material possessions essential in early marriage and unwillingness to assume financial responsibilities;
8. marriage as a threat to career attainment; and
9. occupational isolation precluding contact with the opposite sex (e.g., particularly affecting women in sex-linked occupations such as teaching, nursing, social work, etc.).

For the most part, these attributes profile misfits with personal and/or interpersonal characteristics that might make them candidates for rejection or selection out of marriage. Kuhn suggests that the "rejected type" theory may help explain why some persons never marry but goes on to add that some people fail to marry because of *chance* factors and then as they grow older develop undesirable personality traits resulting from their bitterness over failure to marry. Using this line of reasoning, it is impossible for the unmarried to escape negative labels. If negative characteristics do not preclude their "failure" to marry, then they may develop undesirable attributes as a result of not marrying.

Given the early harsh judgments of the failure to marry or to remain married and subsequent reasons provided as explanations for nonmarriage, perhaps it is not surprising that strong promarriage values were reflected in the developmental tasks designated for young adulthood in the not too distant past. These tasks, of course, carried long-range implications for the family in old age as well. In keeping with earlier values, the developmental tasks for young adulthood underscored the centrality of marriage and the family in definitions of appropriate adult development. Havighurst (1972:2) maintained that "developmental tasks of life . . . are those things that constitute healthy and satisfactory growth in our society." If these tasks are not successfully performed at a particular period of time, then the individual is expected to be unhappy, experience difficulty with later tasks, and encounter social disapproval.

Life-cycle stage models then assume that development is hierarchical, cumulative, and sequenced in time (Stein, 1981). The concept of life stages implies that (a) all normal adults will pass through the stages; (b) accompanying each stage are tasks that must be performed during that period of time; (c) persons are more or less successful in managing crises attendant to accomplishing tasks at given stages; (d) successful resolution of subsequent stages is contingent on successful performance in prior stages; and (e) stages are tied to chronological age (Brim, 1977).

In keeping with a marriage-oriented society, the tasks specified for early adulthood forecast thwarted personal growth and development for persons committed to singlehood as a way of life. The first four tasks—selecting a mate, learning to live with a marriage partner, starting a family, and rearing children—specify aspects of marriage and family as representing "healthy and satisfactory" growth. In accounting for some change, Havighurst (1972:85), however, did allow that "the task of finding a marriage partner is hard to describe as a single definite task of Americans in the 1970s. Few of the rules that seemed stable in the early part of the twentieth century now apply." Yet, change may not be so widespread as projected by Havighurst because marriage remains a highly valued lifestyle by the majority of adults in the United States (Thornton & Freedman, 1983), and more than 90 percent anticipate they will marry and have a lasting marriage. "Having a good family life" continues to be the most important social value for Americans (Gallup, 1982). It is sometimes conveyed that the unmarried do not have a family life. With these values and goals forming a part of the social context in which marital status is evaluated, the atypical, nonnormativeness of singleness is still apparent. But are attitudes changing toward those who may choose to pursue a more marginal status?

CONTEMPORARY ATTITUDES TOWARD SINGLENESS

Only a little over a decade ago and echoing the earlier tie between singleness and the presumed need for supervision of the unmarried despite age, the association between marriage and adulthood continued to be reaffirmed; marriage and "the birth of the first child marks full entrance into adult roles" (Kimmel, 1974:199). "One who is not married, even as biological age increases, tends to be viewed as 'not really grown up.'" Deciding not to marry and not to have children, with the former usually expected to occur first, represent a rejection of perhaps the most pervasive expectations for adults of both sexes. "Indeed, marriage is often projected as the only 'normal' sex role behavior for females" (Havens, 1973:213). Thus, in addition to its being a mark of maturity, marriage fulfills gender roles as well (Duberman, 1977:100).

Consequently, being unmarried whether never married, divorced, or separated violates traditional and apparently continuing expectations for both men and women. The strong expectations for marriage have led to devaluation of singleness and negative stereotypes of the unmarried. In response to what he viewed as the intense societal pressures to marry and the reference to singles as "those who fail to marry" by social scientists as well as others, Stein (1976:4) observed that "The possibility that some people might actually choose to be single because they want to be, because they feel it would contribute to their growth and well-being to remain so, is simply not believed possible." Stein (1976) concluded that singleness for either sex implies belonging to one of two stereotyped groups: the "swingers" or the "lonely losers," although on balance unmarried women are more often seen as objects of sympathy than are single men.

A number of complex factors may figure into the decision to remain unmarried or become single again. Stein (1976) described factors that might move a person from one situation as "pushes" and those that might draw a person toward a situation as "pulls." Pulls toward marriage include, among others, emotional attachment and desire for a family whereas pushes toward marriage and away from singleness could include loneliness, guilt over singleness, and pressure from parents or others. Feeling trapped in a marriage, limited mobility, and lack of new experiences may be pushes toward being single while career opportunities, autonomy, and independence are pulls toward singleness. Depending on their content, attitudes toward nonmarriage may also represent pushes or pulls toward marriage or singleness.

Given the increasing numbers of men and women who are responding to the pulls of nonmarriage and electing to remain single longer or to become single again, how favorable are attitudes toward singleness? In contrast to earlier views of singleness as extreme deviance even among some social scientists (Kuhn, 1948), perhaps finding in a public opinion poll in the late 1970s that 75 percent of respondents regarded being unmarried as "normal" might be seen as representing a shift toward approval. In fairness, it should be noted that much of the early evidence for negative evaluations of the unmarried by the public was based largely on anecdotal information; however, some research provides empirical substantiation for the continuing negative stereotypes of the unmarried (Etaugh & Malstrom, 1981; Wakil, 1980). Cargan and Melko (1982) assessed the accuracy of stereotypes of the unmarried. Although Cargan and Melko found little support for the validity of many of the stereotypes about single people, nevertheless, Etaugh and Malstrom observed that the married were viewed most favorably on more characteristics than any unmarried group. Of the unmarried, the widowed were rated most positively whereas the never married were evaluated more favorably than the divorced who were seen as less dependable, more troubled, and less stable. In their comparison of widowed and divorced, Kitson, Lopata, Holmes, and Meyerling (1980) concluded that divorce remains a stigmatized status. Furthermore, this stigma is apparently internalized by older, divorced women who feel alienated, restricted in their social relationships, and victims of discrimination because of their marital status. This and other evidence point to the extreme salience of marital status as a stimulus to which others respond in social interaction. Marital status, for example, was a greater determinant of the way persons were perceived by others than their gender (Etaugh & Malstrom, 1981).

The negative stereotypes of singles and the difficulties of maintaining a status with little normative and institutional support may erode the self-esteem of the unmarried. Self-esteem is formed from interaction with others and through interpretation of the responses of others. In a marriage, evaluations of partners are salient in determining the self-esteem of one another (Schafer, Keith & Lorenz, 1984) so that marriage has been described as a significant validating relationship for adults (Berger & Kellner, 1975). Not only do singles lack the potentially validating relationship of marriage, but the kind of transitions they experience may be ambiguous, little understood, and perhaps judged harshly. In the unmarried cohort now 65 years of age or older, transitions to singleness were probably more difficult with less peer or institutional support than is found now. When the cohort represented in this book were young, popular articles on single life were written exclusively by or about never-married women with no explicit mention of the problems of never-married or divorced men or of divorced or widowed women (Cargan & Melko, 1982). The normality of marriage was taken for granted. The dynamics of the transition to permanent singleness are poorly understood. Although Wakil (1980) observed less negative attributions to the never married than in the 1950s, role transitions resulting in singleness, whether becoming widowed, divorced or deciding never to marry, seemingly still have as their conclusion a decline in status.

ROLE TRANSITIONS AND SINGLENESS

Types of Transitions to Singleness

Marriage is described as a critical role transition. And research has examined marital roles and factors that contribute to satisfaction and adjustment of both younger and older couples (Brubaker, 1983; Keith & Schafer, 1986). With the exception of studies of widowhood, however, there is limited research on the role transitions and adjustment of the unmarried in old age. Yet, singles undergo transitions in becoming and/or remaining unmarried. They, too, engage in role making and role taking from which they presumably experience benefits, conflict, and role strain as they manage their unmarried status over the life cycle. Role changes, for example, from single to married to single again involve unambiguous rites of passage, but for the never married there also may be transitions in definitions of singlehood in relation to its permanency and the extent of control over the status. And the perceived permanency of the status as well as control over past and future transitions may be salient to adjustment. Furthermore, the degree of permanency and control over marital status may vary across the life cycle and by sex.

Stein (1978) developed a fourfold typology based on the extent to which singleness is voluntary or involuntary and permanent or impermanent. This typology is important because it incorporates elements of selectivity (voluntary-involuntary) and reactions to singleness (preferences for change or remaining the same). Voluntary-stable singles choose singleness with no intention to marry or remarry. This group includes the never married who are satisfied and the widowed or divorced who prefer not to remarry. It also includes members of religious orders whose vocation precludes marriage.

In contrast to one another, the involuntary-stable single and the involuntary-temporary single both may desire marriage, but the latter still expects to marry whereas the former defines singleness as a permanent status. The involuntary-stable group includes older widowed, divorced, or never-married persons who really want to marry, but, unable to find a spouse, they may have come to terms with singleness as a likely outcome for them for the remainder of their lives. Involuntary-temporary singles may be both young and old. Some are young never marrieds who are very interested in marriage or older men and women who want to marry for the first time or to remarry.

The voluntary-temporary single has chosen singleness but intends to marry in the future. For this group at the present time, other interests may eclipse those of seeking a mate.

Just as it is possible to conceptualize marital careers over the life course, we can also identify career patterns in singleness as individuals move from one type to another. Some types may be more prevalent at certain stages of the life cycle. Among the never married, for example, an involuntary-temporary single in youth may end life as a voluntary-permanent single. As persons move from one status to another, however, marriage may or may not intervene in the transition. A voluntary-stable single may have married, divorced, and prefer not to marry again.

The never married also are involved in transitions. No public rite of passage recognizing a new status, however, accompanies the decision for voluntary-permanent singleness. Nevertheless, the assumption that the perceived degree of permanency of the never-married status may fluctuate over the life cycle is implicit in the sterotypes applied to those who have not yet married. For example, persons (especially women) who have not married by a generally unspecified chronological age are viewed as no longer marriageable and in earlier years were described as "on the shelf."

Singles and their significant others, however, may or may not hold congruent definitions of the status of the unmarried. Friends, peers, and family may "pressure" a single toward marriage who subjectively defines his/her status as voluntary and stable. When the transition to permanency occurs, it may be, in large part, a private event. Resulting divergence in expectations between singles and their significant others would seem to contribute to role strain or difficulty in performing a role. Roles of singles are ambiguous (Berk, 1977), and incongruent perceptions of permanency and voluntarism in the role enhance the lack of clarity.

Shifts in conceptions of singleness from voluntary to involuntary or temporary to permanent also may involve stress and strain. We can speculate about what some of the problematic changes may be. It would seem that if individuals desire change but involuntarily occupy a status or role with few or no prospects for a transition, then this would be a source of great strain. For some persons, widowhood or divorce/separation in middle and later life may represent such a circumstance. To others, however, what was initially an involuntary status may come to be viewed positively and its continuance become voluntary.

A number of factors may influence the ease with which singles make transitions in marital status. These dimensions may also be important in determining responses to the various transitions to singleness including those that are accomplished publicly or those undertaken privately.

Correlates of Role Transitions

Control is one of the salient dimensions in determining the ease with which status and role transitions are made. The greater control a person has over a transition, the easier the adjustment to the change. The single who has a choice between singlehood and marriage and elects permanent singleness should make the transition easier than the individual with no opportunities for marriage and who experiences discontinuity in moving from what was viewed as a temporary status to a permanent situation. The latter would encounter their own disappointment and frustration as well as that of significant others at their failure to conform to dominant norms. Austrom and Hanel (cited in Austrom, 1984) demonstrated the importance of individuals feeling that their marital status was voluntary and something over which they had some control. Persons who believed their singleness was due to chance or to circumstances beyond their control were less satisfied with their marital status, with friendships (number and type), with their free time, and they subsequently experienced more relational difficulties than their peers who regarded their marital status as voluntary.

Control over marital status varies across the life cycle. As the number of potential marriage partners diminishes or as individuals take on obligations that may make them less likely to desire marriage or to be seen as marriageable, then they may have less control over the decision to remain single. Geographical location and occupational placement have some effect on opportunities for marriage whereas in middle and later life the disproportionate sex ratio and the increased possibility of poor health also would reduce control over marital status.

Anticipatory socialization facilitates role transitions and role performance (Burr, 1972) and serves notice that roles are expected and intended. In contrast to marriage, singleness is seldom a target of socialization. With the pervasive pressure to marry in our culture, there is little reason to expect that anticipatory socialization for singleness as a permanent status would be likely to occur. Skills for managing singleness must be derived through some means other than early socialization or not at all. The absence of previous socialization will make adaptation to a status more difficult and produce greater role strain.

Timing of change can mitigate the impact of a transition if it is on-time or aggravate the discontinuity if it is off-time (Seltzer, 1970). Transitions in the life course are usually expected to happen at certain points, for example, completion of school, entrance into the labor force, marriage, widowhood in later life, and so on. When life events occur off-time, they require greater effort to adjust.

Nonoccurrence of an expected event (e.g., failure to marry or remarry) however, requires management and adjustment as well. Failure to undergo role changes in the expected direction at the anticipated time entails realignment. Nevertheless, as opportunities for marriage diminish for older singles, the decision for permanent singleness may seem more appropriate and on-time than it would have earlier in the life cycle. Presumably with dissemination of information about the great probability of widowhood, older women can begin to prepare for this transition. Furthermore, such a transition will be expected by significant others. In contrast, the younger never married who voluntarily decide early in life not to marry or perhaps young widows not planning to remarry will have less social support.

They less often have peers in a similar status or support from family members. With increased delays in age at first marriage and/or perhaps nonmarriage for many, opportunities for support from likeminded others should increase in the future.

The salience or importance of a role may determine the amount of strain associated with changes that occur off-time. Marital and family roles are among the most, if not the most, central life roles. Pervasiveness or the degree to which a role influences many aspects of life is salient in increasing the amount of stress encountered when events are off-time or do not occur at all. Singleness traditionally has been conceived as having a pervasive and largely negative influence on life circumstances including finances, physical and mental health, and social relationships (Figure 1.1). And the greater influence of marital status over gender in determining the responses of others (Wakil, 1980) contributes evidence for the extensive and pervasive impact.

Although structural characteristics of role transitions (e.g., amount of control over changes, anticipatory socialization, timing, and salience of the role) may figure in easing transitions, there are also psychological strategies that assist in managing a deviant status such as singleness.

Psychological Strategies for Coping with a Deviant Status

Coming to terms with singleness and maintaining oneself in a deviant status is not unlike the process of legitimating childlessness. Veevers (1975) suggests a variety of defense mechanisms that are used to counter social pressures against childlessness and to sustain a status that is negatively sanctioned. These techniques may also be used in the management and legitimation of singleness although some are clearly more credible at certain times in the life cycle than at others. Thus, not only are structural correlates of role transitions that determine the level of strain accompanying changes age-linked but also the effectiveness of psychological processes for legitimating a deviant status is related to place in the life course.

Persons occupying a deviant status (e.g., singleness or childlessness) may reject that there are differences between them and the persons who are not "deviant" (e.g., married with children or unmarried). That is, in the case of the childless women, they sought to minimize any differences between them and mothers and relied on the possibility of adoption in the future to further reduce the incongruence

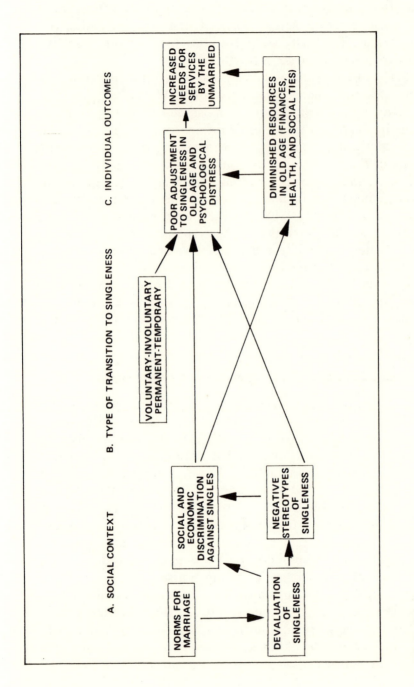

Figure 1.1
Factors Associated with Singleness in Old Age

Reprinted with permission of Baywood Publishers. Keith, P. "The Social Context and Resources of the Unmarried in Old Age." *International Journal of Aging and Human Development*, 1986, 23: 81–96.

(Veevers, 1975). In the same way to minimize the discrepancy between the single and the married, the single may project the possibility of marriage at a future time. Use of this process to resolve dissonance resulting from childlessness and singleness, however, seems highly age-linked; beyond certain ages the likelihood of changing either status diminishes, thus, this mechanism would cease to have much credibility at some points in the life cycle. For example, chances for marriage especially for women decline sharply after age 30, whereas in much the same way, adoption agencies prefer younger couples.

Another strategy is to accept the difference between marriage and singleness but define one's single status as more desirable. This entails evaluating marriage in negative terms. The "pushes" toward singleness identified by Stein (1976) represent negative characteristics of marriage that enable the individual to accept a deviant status and assign a more positive value to it.

Marriage could be perceived as restrictive, boring, stifling, diminishing the possibilities for new relationships, and reducing opportunities for personal development and fulfillment. Veevers (1975) suggests that the process of selective perception is employed by focusing primarily on values that are congruent and supportive of one's beliefs about a deviant status. Evidence can be marshalled either to support marriage or degrade it. Individuals may selectively single out a "bad" marriage for comparison with their single status just as the childless couple may reaffirm the wisdom of their decision when they see a child have a tantrum in a retail store.

Differential association with others who have similar joys and difficulties and are attempting to maintain a comparable status should be another source of support. Organized groups dedicated to singles or at least reaffirming singleness, if not the stereotypic lifestyle of the single as "swinging" and carefree, may also provide support for some. There is probably more support for singles than for the childless; however, some of the commercial appeals to singles almost seem to take advantage of the isolation and vulnerability of younger persons in particular who may be only beginning to develop an ideology of singleness or who may still be regarding it as a way station to marriage hoping to use some of the organizations as a way to meet potential marriage partners. Certainly the growth of age-segregated centers for older persons, many of whom are unmarried, provides an avenue to establish social relationships that are supportive also.

The relative isolation from individuals whose belief systems are different may help maintain a deviant belief system (Veevers, 1975). The childless may associate with other childless couples while the singles may seek out other unmarried individuals and avoid the company of married persons. Frequently, however, this isolation may be unintentional and undesired, for example, in the instance of the single female who is not entertained at the home of married work colleagues. Another strategy is psychological isolation in which deviants may "protect their belief system by becoming very selective in the persons to whom they choose to reveal their true feelings" (Veevers, 1975:479).

Veevers (1975) also suggests that trial parenthood in which couples borrow babies is often structured in such a way that it reaffirms their decision not to have children. For example, the child's family may be undergoing stress through illness, and so forth, the childless couple's house is not "child-proof," and the trial is doomed to failure. In an analogous way, the never-married may invoke trial marriages under conditions that are less than optimal almost insuring that the experience will make their decision for singlehood appear wise.

The childless may reject those who decry their way of life by interpreting the disapproval as envy. Persons in a deviant status may assume that others who are hostile or who pity them are really jealous of the freedom and other benefits accruing from their status. By redefining disapproval of others into envy, the deviant are able to disregard the advice or admonition of others to marry, for example, or to have children because they assume their advisors do not have their best interests in mind but rather are punitive and want them to share the less fulfilling lifestyle of the majority. There probably is envy among the married for some of the more desirable characteristics attributed to singleness. Even if there is not envy of the single it may be important to the social construction of reality of the deviant to believe such jealousy exists so that they can discredit the arguments of those who would have them conform to the norms.

Any of these processes that may be necessary for persons to maintain a variant lifestyle seem to require more time, energy, and effort than conformity. In this way they offer support for Stein's observation that it is "hard" to be single, or more generally, it is difficult to violate accepted practices and survive. As social values change and singleness becomes more normative and regarded as representing a choice rather than an unintended event, then these mechanisms will be less necessary.

In large part, the outcomes of singleness for the present cohort of unmarried aged not only have been pervasive but also generally negative when compared with circumstances of the married. The discrepant life outcomes for married and single men, and to a lesser extent women, have fostered much speculation in an attempt to account for the differences.

Clearly, many of the factors suggesting that single men occupy a disadvantaged status are interrelated. Single men, compared with their married peers, tend to have higher death rates, have more physical and mental difficulties, are significantly (20 times) more likely to be committed to mental institutions, have higher suicide rates, commit more crimes, are more vulnerable to alcoholism, have lower incomes, and experience greater financial distress (Cargan & Melko, 1982; Gilder, 1974; Hyman, 1983; Stein, 1976, 1981).

At least three alternative explanations have been set forth to account for the poor showing that single men make relative to married men and also with some groups of single women. Although any causal links between marital status and health, social, psychological, and financial difficulties of singles remain unclear, there are competing theories about the ordering of the relationships.

The question has been raised as to whether singleness is conducive to greater physical and psychological disability or whether those who are least able emotionally and psychologically are less likely to marry or to remain married. That is, are pathologies or personality characteristics associated with the unmarried a response to the status or were they the factors that precluded their marrying or remaining married initially? Did these factors play a part in selecting them out of marriage or did they emerge as a consequence of the status? One of the explanations for the disadvantaged circumstances of some of the unmarried—the rejected type or selectivity perspective—follows from these questions.

This view is closely drawn from early stereotypes of singles as misfits by positing that the greater difficulties of the unmarried are the "cause" of or have led to their marital status. Implicit in this is the notion that the unmarried are not married because they have been selected out of the marriage process since they were less fit or possessed characteristics that were in some way deterrents to marriage or to staying married. The selectivity explanation implies that those who marry are well-adjusted and healthy (Austrom, 1984), whereas the never married or formerly married fail to remain so because of personal deficiencies.

Selectivity factors, however, figure differentially in whether men or women marry. Unmarried men compare unfavorably with married men on education, occupational status, and income whereas attainments of single women on these dimensions exceed those their unmarried male and married female peers. Thus the rejected type—selectivity argument is not supported for women (Austrom, 1984). Growing out of this perspective, however, is the assumption that singleness is not freely chosen, is not a conscious decision, and is only incurred when marriage or remaining married is not possible.

A second perspective explaining differences in the quality of life of the married and unmarried most directly emphasizes the benefits derived from marriage by men. This view suggests that many of the difficulties experienced by unmarried men can be attributed to the absence of interpersonal support and intimacy derived from marriage that seems especially beneficial to their married peers. In the most extreme statement of this view, it is contended that marriage is necessary to the survival of men and to live without it is very destructive.

Some have held that in the absence of marriage men become isolated and in instances antisocial (Austrom, 1984). In this perspective it is posited that benefits of marriage include not only expressive but also instrumental support. Proponents of the "benefits" of marriage perspective suggest that not only are single men incapable of developing and maintaining emotionally sustaining support systems but they are ill prepared to meet their domestic needs traditionally provided in marriage.

There are few studies that focus on the direct emotional benefits of marriage. But studies that have taken into account loneliness and living alone indicate that it is premature to conclude that marriage by itself provides social support whereas singleness does not (Austrom, 1984). Indeed, having a significant other may be more important than whether or not this person is a marital partner.

In a third more general view of the disadvantaged status of the unmarried it is suggested that difficulties experienced by singles may be outcomes of interaction in a society that devalues and stigmatizes their status rather than resulting directly from the failure to marry. Figure 1.1 presents a model of how various social factors described earlier in the chapter may interact to produce such outcomes for the unmarried in old age.

The expectations and pressures for marriage posited in the model already have been widely documented as have the devaluation and negative perceptions of singleness. The negative outcomes perhaps have been observed most consistently for men. We can only speculate that the demoralization that directly or indirectly may come from interaction with individuals and institutions (social settings and the workplace) that define the single status as deviant and treat it accordingly takes its toll in perceived inadequacies, unhappiness, and eventual social-psychological deterioration and marginality.

Figure 1.1 provides a framework that is partially tested in later chapters. It is suggested in the model that characteristics of the social context of singleness prevalent during the lifetime of persons who are now old were generally unsupportive of the unmarried in several major life areas ranging from finances to mental health. As indicated in the model, earlier evaluations of singleness may have implications for available resources in later life.

As singleness becomes a more typical pattern, negative labeling of singles and discrimination should diminish, and deficits experienced by some of the unmarried may be reduced. The cohort now aged 65 or over, however, reached adulthood at a time when singleness was not normative and remaining or becoming unmarried (except for widowhood) was often viewed as failure and/or attributed to personality, social, or physical deficits of the individual. The importance of the context in which the current generation of single older persons have aged is evident in the model.

Factors promoting single, independent living are more likely to be eroded in old age. Retirement, poor health, and other age-related changes may reduce mobility, social ties, and autonomy for some, creating difficulties and making singleness less viable in later life (Ward, 1979). As resources diminish, the support system of the family that might provide assistance for the married is likely to be smaller and/or inaccessible to a substantial portion of the unmarried. It is important then to determine which groups of the unmarried are most vulnerable to poor health, financial limitations, social isolation, and diminished psychological well-being. From this perspective the remaining chapters address health status (Chapter 3), health care behavior (Chapter 4), financial circumstances (Chapter 5), and the implications of work and retirement for the unmarried (Chapter 6).

How the unmarried manage their nonwork lives, including sex roles within the household and social ties and activities, as well as changes in them are considered in Chapters 7 and 8, respectively. These are followed by an examination of social relationships of the unmarried in rural and urban areas (Chapter 9). Circumstances thought to place the aged at risk of being more vulnerable to a diminished quality of life, for example, isolation, living alone, and childlessness are studied in Chapter 10. Finally, concluding thoughts about the implications of marital status among the unmarried along with a discussion of factors that contributed to their happiness comprise Chapter 11.

Hyman (1983), in his caution that analysts should "stop the common, crude practice" of treating the widowed, divorced-separated, and never married as one group, is heeded. Furthermore, the outcomes of widowhood, divorce-separation, and lifelong singleness for men and women usually are examined separately.

Characteristics of the Sample and Procedures

2

Data reported in the chapters that follow are drawn primarily from the 1969 and 1979 waves of the Longitudinal Retirement History Study conducted by the U.S. Bureau of the Census for the Social Security Administration. Unless otherwise indicated, these waves of data were used in the statistical analyses. Only selected demographic data are presented in this chapter. Additional characteristics of the respondents are discussed as they are pertinent to the topics of later chapters.

The original national sample contained 11,153 persons aged 58 to 63 in 1969. From this sample, a subsample of unmarried men (n = 375) and women (n = 1,674) interviewed in both 1969 and 1979 were studied. The subsample included 264 never-married women, 157 never-married men, 1,159 widowed women, 104 widowed men, 251 divorced/separated women, and 114 divorced/separated men. These men and women had the same marital status at both interviews. The Retirement History Study includes substantial information on demographic and financial characteristics, employment history, physical health, and a few social-psychological variables. See Irelan (1972) for an extensive description of the sampling plan and the background of the larger study. For convenience, the waves of the study will be referred to as time 1 and time 2. Unless otherwise indicated time 1 and time 2 refer to data obtained in 1969 and 1979.

Data were not available to determine the number of years respondents had been widowed, divorced, or separated prior to the initial

interview. Categories of the divorced and separated were combined
and for convenience in the text they are usually referred to as divorced.

Age, Race, Place of Residence

Of course, all respondents were aged 58 to 63 at time 1, and men
and women did not differ in age (t = .41). Their mean age was a little
over 60 years at time 1. Eighty-seven percent of the men and 86 percent of the women were Caucasian. Paralleling national data, the
majority of these older persons lived in places of 2,500 or larger,
67 percent of the men and 74 percent of the women.

Education

Women had obtained somewhat higher levels of education than
men (t = 3.85, p < .001). Thirty-eight percent of the women and
50 percent of the men had less than a high school education. Twenty
percent of the women and 18 percent of the men had completed
high school. Twenty-four percent of the women and 19 percent of
the men were high school graduates whereas 10 percent of the women
and 6 percent of the men had some college. About equal proportions
of men and women were college graduates or had some graduate
education (6 and 7 percent, respectively).

Employment Status

At time 1, 67 percent of the men and 57 percent of the women
were employed. By the end of the decade only 14 and 12 percent of
the total sample of unmarried men and women, respectively, remained
employed.

Income

Income in 1970 was coded into 14 categories ranging from under
$1,000 (1) to $25,000 (14). Income at time 2 was coded into 23 categories ranging from under $1,000 (1) to $30,000 and over (23). The
median income for men at time 1 was in the range of $3,500 to
$3,999 and $2,500 to $2,999 for women. Incomes of men at time 1
were significantly higher than those of women (t = 5.23, p < .001).
At time 2, median incomes of men were in the $4,000 to $4,999

range and were still higher than those of women (\$3,500–\$3,999; $t = 3.63$, $p < .001$).

Occupation

Occupation was coded in 11 categories ranging from laborers to professional, technical, and kindred workers. Other categories included farm laborers, service workers, private household workers, operatives, craftsmen (foreman and kindred workers), sales workers, clerical workers, managers, farmers, and farm managers. Despite their lower incomes, women tended to occupy somewhat higher level occupations than did men ($t = 2.77$, $p < .01$).

Marital Status, Education, and Occupation

Marital status was not related to educational level among men ($F = 1.67$). Never-married men, however, were or had been in higher level occupations than those of divorced men ($F = 5.11$, $p < .01$). Never-married women had completed more education ($F = 29.74$, $p < .001$) and had been in higher level occupations than divorced or widowed women ($F = 21.19$, $p < .001$).

Statistical Models and Tests

The analyses reported in subsequent chapters are considered exploratory and are used to test hypotheses suggested in an often limited body of literature. In keeping with the exploratory nature of the analyses, the .10 level of significance is reported. Analyses of variance and general linear statistical models, including multiple regression and discriminant analyses, were used to examine the link between marital status, gender, and various resources and outcomes.

Initially frequencies, percentages, and, when appropriate, chi square tests were calculated for marital status and for the various resources. One-way analyses of variance were used to test the differences between means by marital status, and t-tests were employed for bivariate analyses of gender. Unless otherwise indicated, the Least Significant Difference test was applied to assess significant differences between means.

In instances in which the dependent variable could be considered a continuous measure, multiple regression models, using ordinary least squares estimation, were fit to the data. Sometimes hierarchical analyses were employed with background variables and interaction terms forming separate blocks. The standardized partial regression coefficients are presented to indicate the net effects of the various independent variables in the equation. The total variance accounted for by variables in the equations is indicated. In hierarchical models, the R^2 attributable to each block is usually reported. When they were available, time 1 levels of the dependent variables were included in the prediction equations. In the hierarchical models, it was possible to assess the relative explanatory power of a block of variables as well as the relative predictive capability of individual factors.

In multivariate analyses in which the dependent variable was categorical, as in the instance of postponement of health care (Chapter 4), the typology of isolation/satisfaction (Chapter 10), and living arrangements (Chapter 10), multiple discriminant analyses were used. Chi square values as tests of significance and canonical correlations are reported. The coefficients from the discriminant analysis are standardized partial regression coefficients that are comparable to standardized coefficients yielded by a multiple regression analysis. In the analyses here, coefficients for the independent variables indicate the relative discriminating power of each factor when others specified in the model are examined. In all instances, bivariate statistics, breakdown tables, and analyses of variance were used to amplify and clarify the interpretation of findings obtained from the discriminant analyses.

In many of the analyses, regression equations were fit separately for gender/marital status subsamples. This procedure permitted an assessment of the relative differences in the patterns of the salient variables for the subgroups. In some analyses, when differences between subgroups were minimal, the total sample or the formerly married were grouped with marital status included as a dummy variable. The multiple regression analysis of health status in the next chapter is an example. Subsample groups, statistical tests, and measures used are clearly identified in each chapter.

Sex, Marital Status, and Health　　　**3**

Health along with income is one of the massive situational factors that affects the lives of older persons (Streib & Schneider, 1971). In fact, health status is used as an indicator of the aging process, and biological changes occurring with age are manifested in health conditions (Hickey, 1980). Generally health problems increase with age although chronic conditions are more prevalent than acute illnesses. Since health has implications for social and psychological well-being, health and health behavior of these unmarried men and women was examined in some detail.

The primary objectives of this chapter were to consider how health conditions and health behavior varied by sex and marital status. To reflect several dimensions of health of the unmarried, a variety of indices was used including presence of a handicap or physical condition that limited mobility and work or housework; physician visits; hospitalization; change in health; and comparison of health with that of others. A multivariate analysis was conducted to identify personal resources that may predict health conditions of the unmarried. Finally, in the next chapter, since postponement of health care is little studied and may figure prominently in the development and progression of chronic problems of the aged, factors that were linked with delay or neglect of health care were identified.

Robbyn Wacker assisted with this chapter.

HEALTH OF THE UNMARRIED

Given increased longevity and its persistent association with gender among older Americans, researchers have examined differences in various aspects of health and health behavior of men and women. Along with gender differences other factors such as living arrangements, marital status, and social networks have been studied in relation to health (Lawton, Moss, & Kleben, 1984; Baldassare, Rosenfield, & Rook, 1984). Although women and men have similar perceptions of the condition of their own health, overall objective health status varies by sex. Women usually report more health problems than men do, but the number mentioning at least one difficulty differs little by sex (Gee & Kimball, 1987). Data from national health surveys indicate that women over 65, for example, experience more days of restricted activity and report more difficulty in physical activities involving mobility than their male counterparts (Verbrugge, 1984). Yet it is more common for men to be unable to perform a major activity (Gee & Kimball, 1987). Whereas women are more frequently ill with both chronic and acute conditions and have more injuries than older men, a larger percentage of men report that they have more total restricted activity days per condition of illness (Verbrugge, 1984). Men are less frequently ill, but their problems are more life threatening than those experienced by women although the latter display more sick role behaviors.

Research that differentiates all categories of marital status in relation to sex and health is somewhat limited since studies have focused more on health of the married and widowed with less attention to the divorced/separated and never married. Older unmarried persons as a group tend to rate their general physical health somewhat poorer than do the married. Some health behavior may also vary by marital status. Verbrugge (1984), for example, found that widowed persons go to the doctor and to the hospital more often than married persons.

Finding differences in morbidity among the unmarried, Verbrugge (1979) concluded that among the noninstitutionalized the divorced and separated are least healthy followed by the widowed and never married. The divorced and separated experience more acute health problems and more limiting chronic conditions. Loss of a spouse, regardless of the type of loss (death or dissolution), is associated with poorer health over time. In a longitudinal study of lower income elderly, Fenwick and Barresi (1981) found that those who lost a spouse through death, divorce, or separation, regardless of when the loss occurred, had lower levels of health than did the married or never married. In taking a somewhat different approach to assessing health status, Lawton et al. (1984) analyzed the relationship between health status, living arrangements, and various measures of well-being. It was concluded that the health status and cognitive measures of well-being of the never married were not different from those of other marital statuses, and those who lived alone were in better health than the unmarried who lived with others.

Based on an extensive review of the literature, Stroebe and Stroebe (1983) found the effect of loss of a spouse on health was greatest among the younger widowed and declined with age. In response to widowhood, women experienced higher rates of reactive depression, mental illness in general, and physical illness. Comparisons of widowers with married men and widows with married women, however, indicated that widowers were worse off than widows relative to their married peers. Thus, Stroebe and Stroebe concluded that the effect of loss of a spouse had a more deleterious effect on the health of widowers than of widows relative to their same-sex married counterparts.

Examining a variety of health indices in relation to marital status, Verbrugge (1979) observed that women were more sensitive to marital status than were men and that marital dissolution had a more negative effect on women in contrast to the conclusion of Stroebe and Stroebe. Separated women followed by divorced women were the most disadvantaged in terms of health compared with married women. Possible reasons for the apparent disparity in the conclusions about the differential effect of marital status on the health of men and women might be because of differences in the quality of data, the range of marital statuses studied, and ages of samples. Research on which Stroebe and Stroebe based their conclusion was limited to secondary analyses of studies of widowhood, which tends to be more prevalent among older persons. Whereas Verbrugge's research covered a wider range of ages and was based on pooled data from national samples, Stroebe and Stroebe commented on the weakness of their sources of data. Finally, the conclusions of Stroebe and Stroebe were drawn from within sex comparisons for married versus widowed but Verbrugge employed both within and between sex comparisons for multiple categories of the unmarried. Certainly differences in previous findings and limitations of data regarding

marital status, gender, and health highlight the need for further investigation. In the sections that follow relationships between indices of
health and gender among the unmarried are examined.

HEALTH LIMITATIONS ON MOBILITY

Respondents indicated whether they had a health condition, physical handicap, or disability that limited their ability to get around. At
time 1, 26 percent of the sample had a health limitation. But by the
end of the decade, 42 percent had a handicap or limitation.

Although Verbrugge (1984) found that women have more problems with mobility than men, these unmarried men and women did
not differ significantly in their handicaps or disabilities that limited
mobility at time 1 ($\chi^2 = 1.09$) or time 2 ($\chi^2 = 1.07$). Corresponding
to data from national surveys, however, divorced/separated men were
most likely to have activities limited by a handicap or disability
(53 percent), although fewer widowed (38 percent) and never-married
men (39 percent) had these limitations by the end of the decade
($\chi^2 = 6.29$, p $<$ .05). Physical limitations had increased among
divorced men over the decade by more than 20 percent compared
with about 12 percent for widowed and never married.

Marital status was associated with the presence of handicaps or
disabilities among women at both interviews ($\chi^2 = 15.16$, p $<$ .001;
11.60, p $<$ .01). At time 1, over one-third of the divorced women
had a handicap or disability that limited their getting around, with
somewhat fewer of the widowed (26 percent) and the never married
(19 percent) bothered by these health limitations. By time 2, similar
percentages of widowed (44 percent) and divorced women (46 percent) reported health limitations whereas the never married continued to have fewer problems, although by then over one-third of them
also had health difficulties that curtailed mobility.

INTERFERENCE WITH WORK OR HOUSEWORK

Men and women noted whether their health limited the amount or
kind of work or housework they could do. At time 1, 34 percent
experienced a problem that affected their work, whereas by time 2,
48 percent had problems serious enough that they influenced their
work or functioning in the household. At time 1, men were a little
more likely to report that their health interfered with their work

(40 percent) than were women (33 percent) (x^2 = 5.78, p < .05). However, at the last interview, men and women did not differ in health limitations on work or housework (x^2 = .51) although health difficulties that interfered with work were more prevalent among both men (50 percent) and women (48 percent) than ten years earlier.

Health limitations on the ability to work were not associated with marital status among men at either interview (x^2 = .48; 4.07). Divorced men, however, experienced the greatest increase in health limitations that interfered with work over the decade. At both times, divorced (36 percent; 47 percent) and widowed women (34 percent; 50 percent) were more likely to have experienced health limitations affecting their work or housework than were never-married women (26 percent; 38 percent); x^2 = 7.29, p < .05; 12.83, p < .01. The percentage of widows who were limited in their work had increased the most.

PHYSICIAN CARE

At both times, a majority of the respondents had received care from a physician during the preceding year, although at the end of the decade more persons reported seeing a physician (66 percent vs. 77 percent). At both time 1 and time 2 and paralleling other literature, women (69 percent, time 1; 79 percent, time 2) were a little more likely than men (55 percent; 71 percent) to have received care from a physician (x^2 = 24.11, p < .001; 10.85, p < .001).

Marital status did not affect the use of physician care by men at either time 1 (x^2 = .32) or time 2 (x^2 = 2.52). At the end of the decade, widowed women were most likely to have seen a physician during the preceding year (80 percent), whereas three-fourths of the divorced and never-married women had obtained care (x^2 = 6.46, p < .05).

NUMBER OF PHYSICIAN VISITS

Respondents indicated the number of times they had obtained care from a physician during the year preceding both interviews. Women had made slightly more visits at time 1 ($\overline{X}$ = 10.74) than had men ($\overline{X}$ = 9.22), but they did not differ significantly (t = 1.69, p < .10). Shanas and Maddox (1980) also reported that women were more likely than men to see a doctor outside the hospital setting. At time 2, men had averaged slightly more than 11 physician visits compared with 9 for women (t = 1.06). Of those who had sought care from a physician, the number of physician visits was not differentiated by marital status among men (F = .98; 1.99) or women (F = 2.35; .22) at either interview although divorced men averaged 16 visits compared with 9 for the widowed and never married.

HOSPITALIZATION

Respondents indicated whether or not they had been hospitalized during the preceding year. At time 1, 10 percent had received care in a hospital compared with 17 percent by time 2. Men and women initially did not differ in their use of a hospital (χ^2 = 00). Consistent with other literature (Shanas & Maddox, 1976), at time 2, more men (22 percent) than women (16 percent) had been hospitalized although the differences were small (χ^2 = 7.99, p < .01). There was no relationship between marital status and having been hospitalized during the preceding year for men or women at time 1 (χ^2 = .08; χ^2 = 3.16) or at time 2 for women (χ^2 = .36). At the end of the decade, however, twice as many divorced (30 percent) as widowed men (15 percent) had been hospitalized, whereas 21 percent of the never married men had received inpatient care (χ^2 = 6.77, p < .05).

EFFECTS OF HEALTH LIMITATIONS ON EMPLOYMENT

Respondents with health limitations (n = 148 men and 549 women) indicated whether their health kept them from working altogether. Over one-third (35 percent) of those who had a health limitation found it serious enough to preclude their working. There was no difference by sex in whether health prohibited employment (χ^2 = .11).

Marital status was not related to the inability to work because of health limitations among men (χ^2 = .29) or women (χ^2 = 2.31). Of those who continued to work, however, poor health interfered so that women were less likely (36 percent) than men (69 percent) to work full-time (χ^2 = 32.11, p < .001).

Among men with a health difficulty who continued to work, marital status was not significantly related to the amount of time they could work (χ^2 = 1.86). More widowed women were bothered by health problems that limited them to part-time employment (69 percent) than divorced (48 percent), or never-married women (χ^2 = 10.69, p < .01). These findings contrast somewhat with those of

Verbrugge (1979) who found that formerly married men and women have the highest prevalence of complete and partial work disabilities of all other marital statuses with the strongest effect among men.

CHANGE IN HEALTH

The majority of respondents experienced stable health over the decade. When time 1 and time 2 measures of health limitations on mobility and interference with work or housework were cross-tabulated, the percentage who gave the same evaluation of health at time 1 and time 2 ranged from 60 and 74 percent among the various sex and marital status categories (Table 3.1). Of those who had changed, the largest proportion experienced a decline in health, ranging from 62 to 77 percent. Divorced and never-married women tended to report somewhat more stable health conditions than other groups. However, when women did experience changes, they, along with divorced men, more often tended to have negative changes in health (Table 3.1).

Table 3.1
Change in Health Condition and Comparisons by Sex and Marital Status

A. Change in Health Condition that Restricted Mobility, Time 1, Time 2		Percent of Those who Changed	
	% Stable	% Change	% Improve	% Decline
Men				
Widowed	69	31	31	69
Divorced	60	40	24	76
Never Married	69	31	31	69
Women				
Widowed	66	34	23	77
Divorced	73	27	29	71
Never Married	74	26	23	77

Table 3.1 (continued)

B. Change in Health Condition that Limited Work or Housework, Time 1,
    Time 2 by Sex and Marital Status

			Percent of Those who Changed	
	% Stable	% Change	% Improve	% Decline
		Men		
Widowed	65	35	36	64
Divorced	68	32	25	75
Never Married	68	32	38	62
		Women		
Widowed	66	34	25	75
Divorced	74	26	29	71
Never Married	70	30	29	71

C. Change in Comparison of Health at Time 1, Time 2 by Sex and
    Marital Status

			Percent of Those who Changed	
	% Stable	% Change	% Improve	% Decline
		Men		
Widowed	61	39	41	59
Divorced	45	55	53	47
Never Married	48	52	48	52
		Women		
Widowed	52	40	50	50
Divorced	58	42	49	51
Never Married	60	40	50	50

COMPARISON OF HEALTH WITH OTHERS

At both interviews respondents reflected on whether their health was better, worse, or the same as that of other people their age. At the first interview, the majority indicated that their health was the same (43 percent) or better (39 percent) than that of their age peers. About equal percentages rated their health as poorer than that of others at both beginning and end of the decade (19 percent and 17 percent, respectively). The percentage who evaluated their health as better than that of others declined only slightly over the decade from 39 percent to 36 percent whereas persons who viewed their health as similar to that of others increased from 43 to 47 percent.

Marital status was not related to comparisons of health among men at either interview (F = 2.20; F = .86). Among women, the never married estimated their health to be better than that of their age peers more often than the formerly married at both interviews (F = 3.13, p < .05; F = 3.29, p < .05). Never-married men did not share this position relative to their peers. Even so, differences among the groups of women were small.

CHANGES IN COMPARISONS OF HEALTH

Comparisons of health with that of others were less stable than evaluations of health limitations. The proportion of those who had not changed their assessments ranged from 45 to 61 percent (Table 3.1). Divorced and never-married men had the least consistent comparisons. In general, women changed their evaluations somewhat less than men although the differences were not great. Except for divorced men, a slight majority of those who had changed their assessments believed that their health had declined relative to that of others. Widowed men, who had the most stable evaluations, also were most likely to have maintained more negative appraisals over the decade.

MULTIVARIATE ANALYSIS OF HEALTH

Health at time 2 was examined in a multivariate analysis of the total sample in which health at time 1 was controlled, and demographic characteristics were added as a second block of variables. Interaction terms for sex and marital status and sex and race were included as a third group of variables. Marital status was represented by two variables; in Mar 1, widowed and never married were coded

Table 3.2

Hierarchical Multiple Regression Analysis of Health (Time 2) for Total Sample

	r	Beta (Model I)	Beta (Model II)	Beta (Model III)
Health (Time 1)	.41	.41**	.37**	.37**
Age	-.05		-.03	-.02
Sex	.01		.02	-.08
Race	-.06		.00	.01
Income	.19		.08**	-.02
Education	.10		-.03	-.03
Employment status	.19		.12**	.12**
Marital Status 1 (Mar 1)	-.04		-.00	-.20**
Marital Status 2 (Mar 2)	.08		.06**	-.07
Sex x Income	.19			.12
Sex x Mar 1	-.03			.19**
Sex x Mar 2	.09			.12
Increase in R^2			.025	.002
R^2		.166	.192	.194

*p <.10

**p <.05

as 0 and divorced as 1. In Mar 2, widowed and divorced were coded
as 0 and never married as 1. Health was measured by combining the
two items on health conditions describing the extent to which health
limited mobility and restricted work/housework. A higher score indicated better health.

Nineteen percent of the variance in health was explained, but most
of it was accounted for by health at time 1 (Table 3.2). Employment
status was significantly associated with health indicating those still in
the labor force enjoyed better health. Other research has demonstrated that those who classify themselves as usually working, perceive
themselves to be in better health (Department of HEW, 1978). Testing

a multivariate model revealed that the divorced also tended to have poorer health than the widowed and never married. When other variables were controlled, a significant sex by marital status interaction effect showed that divorced men had the poorest health although this interaction explained little variance. Thus, after removing the effect of health at time 1, demographic characteristics contributed little to the explanation of health later in life. The lack of demographic explanations of health status found in this study departs somewhat from other literature. For example, others have reported a correlation between lower socioeconomic status and poor health (Shanas & Maddox, 1976). In addition, race has also been found to be associated with marginal health status, with whites benefiting from better health than nonwhites (Shanas & Maddox, 1976).

SUMMARY AND DISCUSSION

The majority of these unmarried men and women had enjoyed stable health over the decade. Limitations on mobility and interference with work or housework had not increased precipitously for most. When health status changed, however, it most often declined. Health behavior also changed somewhat over the ten years in that by the end of the decade these unmarried more often had seen a physician during the preceding year than earlier and had been hospitalized.

Positive evaluations of health were reflected in favorable comparisons of their health with that of age peers. At both the beginning and end of the decade more than 80 percent believed their health was the same or better than that of other older persons. This may reflect some adjustment in assessments on the part of those with poor health because they may accept limitations as normative and evaluate their health the same as that of peers. Or persons may regard their own health appreciatively despite chronic difficulties.

Sex was not a very important factor in differentiating the ratings of health status or in the health behavior of these unmarried. Of the 11 tests (5 indices of health or health behavior X 2 interviews plus 1 test at time 1 only), four tests revealed somewhat different experiences for men and women. However, having sought care from a physician in the last year, which was more characteristic of women, was the only health dimension for which there was a significant sex difference at both interviews. Verbrugge (1985) also found that women obtain help from physicians more often than men. Later in their lives, however, more of these unmarried men than women had been hospitalized during the preceding year perhaps indicating the greater severity of their illnesses.

Likewise, marital status failed to differentiate several measures of health status and behavior with much consistency. When there were differences, however, the divorced fared least well on some of the most critical dimensions indicating health problems. Divorced men, for example, had more limitations on mobility, were hospitalized more, and experienced more negative changes in health conditions compared to other men. Divorced women had more health limitations on mobility and interference with work and housework consistently over the decade than never-married women.

Finally, health enjoyed by the unmarried was largely independent of objective socioeconomic characteristics (e.g., education, income) although being employed was associated with better health. To the extent there were differences, the divorced, especially men, seemed at greater risk of poorer health. A number of factors suggest that divorced/separated men may be more vulnerable to adverse life conditions that may impact health. For example, Hyman (1983) found that their more negative feelings and outlooks on life and society distinguished them from married and widowed men and women, although he did not study the never married. Divorced/separated men are less integrated into the wider world through the use of media or membership in formal organizations, substantially less satisfied with their health and finances (Hyman, 1983), and more vulnerable to alcoholism. They may lead more risk prone lives than widowed or never-married older men. In the next chapter, following up the thought that risk proneness may extend to postponement of treatment, I investigate the extent to which marital status and its relationship to uncertain finances and hardships are linked to a lack of response to health problems.

Postponement of Health Care   4

This chapter investigates one aspect of health behavior of the unmarried—the postponement of needed treatment. To the degree that seeking care without delay may promote health at any age, the reasons people postpone needed care warrants study.

It was recently observed that ". . . willingness to care for health problems has had surprisingly little empirical attention" (Verbrugge, 1985). Determining why persons postpone or delay care is important because preventive measures can reduce the probability of developing chronic disease and disability (Atchley, 1985). Treatment can sometimes reverse the potentially negative effects of chronic disease, and rehabilitation can aid in restoration of lost functions and provide compensation for unrestorable functions. Early detection and prevention of disability should improve the quality of life by both maximizing independence and reducing health care costs (Besdine, 1981). Since the aged and the unmarried use a disproportionate amount of health services and experience more severe chronic illnesses, investigation of why the aged fail to seek needed care should be informative for those providing health services.

There is little available information on the extent of postponement of needed treatment by the aged. In most research, not seeking care when it is warranted is likely included in the general category of nonreported illness or lack of use. Besdine (1981) described the failure of the elderly to report or to conceal illness as a "pervasive behavioral phenomenon." Citing research from Scotland, he suggested that unreported illness may be, in part, responsible for advanced disease states that foster major disability in the frail elderly (Besdine, 1981). Pioneering geriatricians in Scotland found a surprisingly large amount of concealed illness despite free care and accessible physicians. "Non-reporting of symptoms reflecting underlying disease in elderly persons is an especially dangerous phenomenon when coupled with the American organizational structure of health care delivery. Our health care system is passive, especially for elderly people, and lacks prevention-oriented or early detection efforts" (Besdine, 1981). Postponement of care by the elderly increases the probability that disease will be advanced before the person enters the health care system.

Given the importance of seeking care, how prevalent is postponement of treatment? Harris et al. (1981) found that 13 percent of a sample of 1,836 persons age 65 or over had not seen a doctor about their health when they thought they should have (Harris et al., 1981). The most common reason for symptom tolerance and not seeking treatment was expensiveness of care (39 percent) followed by not being sick enough (21 percent), not wanting to bother the doctor (21 percent), and difficulty in getting to the doctor's office or hospital (11 percent). In the Scottish sample, the most frequent explanation for not seeking care was the belief that illness, functional decline, and feeling sick accompany old age and are a normal part of growing older. Depression, intellectual loss, and fear that therapeutic intervention would generate functional loss and impede independent living were additional explanations for not getting treatment (Besdine, 1981). Demographic characteristics that might also may be factors in forgoing care were not reported, although much research has examined them as correlates of use or nonuse of health services (e.g., see Coulton & Frost, 1982).

CORRELATES OF POSTPONEMENT OF HEALTH CARE

Previous research on factors associated with use of health services is instructive for the study of postponement of care although delay in seeking or foregoing needed care may often be categorized with other types of nonuse. Therefore, predictors of postponement of care may have been obscured in research on more general issues of nonuse. Nonuse of health care services, of course, could include those who did not seek assistance because they did not need it along with those who failed to obtain help when it was warranted.

A conceptual approach suggesting that the use of health services is a consequence of predisposing, enabling, and need variables was selected to guide the multivariate analysis of postponement of care in the present research (Anderson & Newman, 1973). Predisposing variables include personal characteristics that may influence perceptions of need or use of services (e.g., demographic characteristics, age, sex), social structural variables (occupation, education, ethnicity), and beliefs about illness and health care. Enabling factors such as income, transportation, and insurance may facilitate or restrain the use of services after need is recognized. Perceived need (individual perceptions of symptoms and self-assessed health) and needs as determined by physicians comprise the need variables.

Predisposing, enabling, and need variables are differentially associated with use of services (Anderson & Newman, 1973; Mechanic, 1979). In general, although there are limited studies of the aged, assessments of need or illness explain more the variance in the use of medical services than social, structural, or psychological factors. It is unclear whether models that explain differential use of services for the general population operate in the same way for unmarried men and women.

In this research, measures representing predisposing, enabling, and need variables were examined in relation to postponement of necessary treatment among the unmarried. Need and enabling variables were represented by self-assessed health and income, respectively. Consistent with the research of Coulton & Frost (1982), social isolation and psychological distress were included as predisposing variables.

Research on the influence of isolation on use of services is somewhat contradictory. Shuval (1970) found that isolates were more likely to secure services perhaps as a substitution for new contacts while Coulton and Frost (1982) observed that the most isolated used the fewest services. Still other research has indicated that large networks of friends prompt seeking health care whereas large family networks support delaying behavior (McKinlay, 1981).

In general, various measures of psychological distress have been linked with increased use of health services (Tessler, Mechanic, & Dimond, 1976). Several reasons for this relationship have been given: (1) distress may be a causal factor in illness; (2) distressed persons may be less skeptical of medical care and believe they have less control over illness; or (3) they may deal with other kinds of problems in their lives by obtaining medical care (Tessler, Mechanic, & Dimond, 1976). Because finances are precarious for many of the unmarried, especially the divorced, perceived financial hardship and comparative financial difficulties were included as assessments of psychological distress. Financial worries and hardships may figure differently from other types of psychological distress in decisions about health care. Harris et al. (1981) found that finances were viewed as a barrier to obtaining care. For this reason, financial distress may diminish use of services and have as a consequence postponement of needed care.

PROCEDURES

Health Care Behavior

To assess whether respondents had postponed health care, they were asked, "Is there some kind of care or treatment that you have put off even though you may still need it? (yes/no). Why have you put it off?" Reasons for postponement were categorized as: financial, convenience, emotional, and "other." Respondents were asked these questions at both time 1 and time 2.

Those who indicated they had not postponed health care may have included both persons who needed care and obtained treatment and those who did not need care and, hence, had not sought it. Data were not available to determine whether a "no" response meant care had been sought or that care was not needed. However, in the multivariate analyses, health status was controlled.

Health

While it is most desirable to have both physician ratings and individual assessments, only self-ratings of health were available. Research, however, has indicated that physician and individual ratings of health are correlated.

The measure of health assessed functional capacity; responses to two questions were summed: "Do you have any health condition, physical handicap, or disability that limits how well you get around?" and "Does your health limit the kind or amount of work or housework you can do?" (yes, 0; no, 1). Health was measured at both time 1 and time 2.

Income

Income for time 1 and time 2 was coded as described in Chapter 2. A higher value indicated higher income.

Distress

Two measures of distress representing predisposing factors were employed in both interviews. Distress over level of living was assessed by asking: "Generally, how satisfied are you with the way you are living now—that is, as far as money and what you are able to have are concerned? Would you say the way you are living is—More than satisfactory (4) to Very unsatisfactory (1)?"

Financial hardship was measured by responses to: "Which of the following four statements describes your ability to get along on your income? I can't make ends meet (1); I have just enough, no more (2); I have enough, with a little extra sometimes (3); I always have money left over (4)."

Isolation

Isolation from both friends and relatives was considered in relation to postponing care. In the earlier interview, respondents indicated the number of friends and relatives whom they contacted in person or by phone "daily, weekly, monthly, less than monthly, or not at all." These were recoded so that scores ranged from 4 (daily contact) to 0 (no contact). At the second interview, persons were asked separate questions about how often they phoned or saw friends or relatives face to face with five response categories ranging from "daily" to "not at all." To correspond more closely to the measure used in the earlier interview, responses were summed for phoning and contact in person; scores ranging from 0 to 4 were obtained for contacts with both friends and relatives.

Analyses

Discriminant analyses were used to determine which combination of factors best differentiated those who had postponed treatment from those who had not. Discriminant function technique identifies the linear combination of variables that best discriminates between discrete groups. Coefficients weighting the variables indicate the relative importance of a factor in the discrimination process and can be interpreted similarly to beta values obtained in multiple regression. In the discriminant analysis, the effect of health status was controlled prior to examination of the remaining variables.

Table 4.1
Postponement and Reasons for Postponement of Health Care by Sex and Marital Status

Men

Marital Status	Postponement (Percentages)		Reasons (Percentages)					
			Financial		Convenience		Emotional	
	Time 1	Time 2	Time 1	Time 2	Time 1	Time 2	Time 1	Time 2
Widowed	31	30	62	52	12	23	15	13
Divorced	25	25	46	54	27	21	18	4
Never Married	22	27	15	17	21	17	27	24
Total Sample	26	29	39	38	21	20	21	15
	$X^2=2.55$, 2 df, ns	$X^2=.76$, 2 df, ns						

Women

Marital Status	Postponement (Percentages)		Reasons (Percentages)					
			Financial		Convenience		Emotional	
	Time 1	Time 2	Time 1	Time 2	Time 1	Time 2	Time 1	Time 2
Widowed	32	31	52	54	17	18	12	14
Divorced	33	27	56	45	22	25	10	18
Never Married	19	21	39	27	22	27	15	39
Total Sample	30	29	51	49	18	20	12	17
	$X^2=17.79$, 2 df, p<.001	$X^2=11.44$, 2 df, p<.01						

RESULTS

Postponement of Health Care

Respondents indicated that if they had put off any medical treatment in the years immediately prior to the interviews. Among the total sample, similar percentages of persons had put off treatment at both times 1 and 2; about 29 percent reported they had postponed treatment at each interview. Men and women did not differ significantly in the frequency with which they had forgone needed care at either time (χ^2 = 2.30, time 1; .58, time 2). The proportion of the unmarried who had not sought needed treatment was more than double that reported by Harris et al. (1981) for a sample of persons 65 years of age or older although no data were presented by marital status or gender.

Marital Status and Postponement of Health Care

Marital status did not figure prominently in the decisions of men to forgo seeking medical care at either time but the widowed were somewhat more likely to delay treatment than the never married at time 1 (Table 4.1). In contrast, marital status was a factor in the decisions of women at both times. Widowed and divorced women failed to obtain needed care more often than the never married both earlier and later in their lives.

Gender and Reasons for Postponement of Care

Respondents indicated why they had put off seeking treatment. Reasons included finances, convenience, and emotional factors. Financial reasons were dominant at both the beginning and end of the decade for both men and women (Table 4.1). However, when the total sample was considered, finances figured in the decisions of women to forego care more often than those of men at both interviews (χ^2 = 7.46, p < .05; χ^2 = 3.86, p < .05). About 40 percent of the men gave finances as reasons compared to one half of the women (Table 4.1).

At time 1, men were more likely to attribute postponement of treatment to emotional reasons than did women (21 percent vs. 12 percent) although they were similar at time 2, 15, and 17 percent respectively. Men and women were about equally likely (around one-fifth) to give convenience as a reason why they did not obtain treatment.

Marital Status and Reasons for Postponement of Care

The relationship between marital status and financial reasons for postponing care was comparable for men and women over time. In general, finances were submitted more often as reasons for delaying care by the widowed and divorced and substantially less frequently by the never married regardless of gender (Table 4.1).

Emotional reasons for delaying care were linked with marital status and, for the most part, never-married men and women were more likely to mention emotional reasons for not obtaining care. For example, at time 2, only 4 percent of the divorced men compared to 24 percent of the never married gave emotional reasons for not securing care and at the second interview, twice as many of the never-married women (39 percent) gave emotional reasons as widowed (14 percent) or divorced (18 percent) women. By time 2, emotional reasons figured more importantly in decisions about care than financial aspects among never-married men and women. Marital status, however, had little effect on decisions based on convenience (Table 4.1).

Change in Postponement of Health Care

In this section, the extent to which the tendency to postpone health care was stable over time was studied. The majority of persons who had postponed treatment at time 1 continued to delay seeking treatment. More than two-thirds of both men and women, regardless of marital status, behaved much the same at both times (Table 4.2). The percentages whose behavior was stable over the decade ranged from 66 percent of the divorced women to 79 percent of the widowed women.

Furthermore, most who did change over the ten years were likely to change negatively and neglect treatment whereas earlier they had sought health care (Table 4.2). Divorced men and women were an exception in that when they changed they were somewhat more likely to seek treatment than their counterparts. Among men, for example, only 40 percent of the widowed and never married who changed obtained treatment compared to 60 percent of the divorced men who elected to seek treatment. The pattern for marital status and

Table 4.2
Change in Postponement of Health Care, Time 1 and Time 2

	% Stable	% Change	% of Those Who Changed	
			% Obtained Treatment	% Postponing Treatment
Marital Status		Men		
Widowed	70	30	42	58
Divorced	69	31	60	40
Never Married	74	26	40	60
		Women		
Widowed	66	34	50	50
Divorced	66	34	59	41
Never Married	79	21	45	55

change in seeking care was comparable for women although differences between the statuses were smaller than for men.

Multivariate Analyses of Postponement of Care

Discriminant analyses were used to assess whether need, enabling, or predisposing variables best differentiated persons who delayed care from those who did not postpone treatment (Table 4.3). Among men the factors discriminated between health care behavior of the divorced best and were least salient for the never married. There was one significant function for widowed and divorced men at time 1 and one for the divorced at time 2. There was one significant function for all groups of women at both time 1 and time 2. Except for widowed women, the variables tended to be somewhat better discriminators of postponement of health care earlier in the lives of the unmarried.

In the majority of instances, either financial hardship or dissatisfaction with level of living were more important determinants of postponement of care than health status. For example, of the 12 tests (2 interviews X gender X 3 marital statuses), health was the most salient factor in only three instances.

For most, distress over level of living or perceived financial hardship had a greater direct effect on delaying care than actual income.

Table 4.3

Factors Related to Postponement of Treatment by Marital Status: Standardized Discriminant Function Coefficients

Factors	Postponement of Treatment											
	Widowed				Divorced				Never Married			
	Men		Women		Men		Women		Men		Women	
	T1	T2	T1	T2	T1	T2	T1	T2	T1	T2	T1	T2
Health	.38	.23	.63	.34	.89	.41	.44	.21	.44	.36	.47	.60
Income	.04	-.32	.14	.08	-.14	-.11	-.03	.06	.74	.63	.33	.31
Financial Hardship	.63	.23	.34	.40	-.11	.88	.10	.29	-.52	.08	-.15	.08
Distress-Level of Living	.15	.88	.20	.57	.41	-.16	.70	.53	.50	.25	.56	.33
Isolation:												
Friends	-.12	.11	.15	.06	.09	.09	-.09	.37	.07	.36	.20	.32
Relatives	.34	.05	.04	-.11	.10	.28	.33	.09	-.11	-.17	-.35	-.08
Canonical Correlation	.42	.32	.29	.29	.57	.33	.40	.25	.28	.25	.36	.32
χ^2 (df = 6)	16.67	10.91	91.10	103.70	35.19	12.72	39.23	16.10	10.99	9.87	31.17	28.75
p	.01	.10	.001	.001	.001	.05	.001	.01	.10	(ns)	.001	.001

Income probably contributed to perceptions of financial difficulties that in turn affected decisions about obtaining care. An exception was never-married men for whom income tended to be associated directly with obtaining care especially at the first interview.

SUMMARY AND DISCUSSION

About 30 percent of these unmarried had not sought care when their health condition warranted it. Furthermore, the tendency to delay care was fairly stable over time. As a group, these unmarried were about twice as likely to delay health care than was observed in another sample of both married and unmarried men and women aged 65 or over (Harris et al., 1981). The unmarried may be more vulnerable to life strains that influence their decisions to obtain care. Compared to another national sample of men and women including married and unmarried (Harris et al., 1981), a higher percentage of these singles had not obtained care because of expense. Finances may have represented a chronic strain for much of the sample, since economic hardship and distress were dominant reasons for postponing care across the decade.

Gender was not a factor in forgoing care although some research suggests that women may be more likely than men to obtain care, and these unmarried women were more apt than men to have seen a physician at least once in the preceding year. Postponement may represent a different dimension of health behavior from use or nonuse. This may be further illustrated in the importance of distress over level of living and financial hardship to postponing care relative to health as a measure of need. Either distress over level of living or financial hardship loomed large in decisions to postpone care by most men and women and were more important than health status for the majority. This contrasts with other research on use/nonuse that has generally found need (health condition) as more salient than predisposing variables, including distress, in determining utilization of services. The discrepancy between these findings and other research may be because in some inquiries postponement of needed treatment is not considered separately from other types of nonuse even though its origins may be quite different. To the degree that finances and distress over economic circumstances may be amenable to intervention and change, then these findings may be of use to professionals as they attempt to increase preventive and followup care.

Marital status differentiated the delaying behavior of women but not that of men with never-married women less likely to forego care than their formerly married peers. Although marital status per se was not linked with postponement among men, it was associated with reasons for delaying treatment for both men and women. A most striking finding was the marked difference between the formerly married and the never married, especially among men, in attributing finances as reasons for delaying care. More than three times as many formerly married men as never married claimed finances as reasons for their health care decisions. The less importance assigned to finances by the never married probably reflected their somewhat better economic situation although never-married women were substantially more constrained by finances earlier in their lives than were men.

Some research has indicated that large networks of friends prompt seeking health care whereas generous family networks support delaying behavior (McKinlay, 1981). By the end of the decade, decisions of divorced women and never-married men and women, somewhat more than those of others, were influenced by friendship connections. Weak ties with friends were linked to postponing care; to address this it may be possible to increase educational and organizational activities that provide opportunities for the unmarried to form social relationships.

By the end of the decade for women and at both points for men, health behavior of the never married was more hindered by emotional reasons. The specific emotional reasons were not identified; presumably they may have included thinking that physicians could not help them, fear of diagnoses, or anxiety about procedures. Whatever their origins, emotional reasons were substantial barriers to obtaining care for women at time 2 and sustained barriers for men over time.

These findings underscore the need for preventive education among the unmarried. The widowed and never married of both sexes who changed their health care behavior over time were more likely to change negatively and postpone treatment than were the divorced. Among the most important findings were that proportions of men and women who neglected to obtain care and their reasons for doing so were fairly stable over time. This indicates there are persistent strains in the lives of older unmarried persons that may be addressed by professionals who are in positions to intervene, provide assistance, and to address barriers to obtaining treatment. Reasons given by the formerly married and never married for not obtaining care indicated somewhat divergent needs that would seem to warrant differential attention by practitioners. The emotional reasons cited by never married are one example. Early intervention might have removed or diminished what became fairly stable obstructions to seeking care by these unmarried over the decade.

Finances of the Unmarried

5

Although research indicates the married fare better financially than the unmarried, it is less clear how finances and subjective evaluations of economic well-being vary among widowed, divorced, and never-married older men and women. The objectives of this chapter are to compare finances and evaluations of finances by sex and marital status among the unmarried at the beginning and end of a decade and to investigate factors associated with satisfaction with level of living and financial hardship for the widowed, divorced/separated, and never married. Despite some lack of clarity on the differential effects of widowhood, divorce/separation, or lifelong singleness on financial circumstances in old age, literature addressing the objective and subjective aspects of finances of the unmarried is instructive.

FINANCES OF THE UNMARRIED AGED

Income

Both unmarried men and unmarried women are especially vulnerable to economic deprivation (Pearlin & Johnson, 1977). Across the life cycle, men and women with spouses present in the household enjoy substantially higher combined family incomes than their unmarried peers (Statistical Abstract of the United States, 1986). Table 5.1, however, shows individual (not family) income by age, sex, and marital status. Sex differences, of course, are evident in the figures for total median income (Table 5.1). In the younger age group

Table 5.1
Individual Median Income by Age, Sex, and Marital Status in 1984

Age	Men					Women				
	Married	Never Married	Widowed	Divorced	Total	Married	Never Married	Widowed	Divorced	Total
25-64	$23,101	$13,733	$12,015	$18,141	$20,934	$7,288	$12,774	$9,134	$12,652	$8,686
65+	11,317	6,833	7,936	6,991	10,450	4,866	8,654	6,568	6,777	6,020

Source: Current Population Reports, Series P-60. Page 114. No. 151, 1986.

(25 to 64 years), men have median incomes of $20,934 compared to $8,686 for women. The same pattern of sex differences exists for persons 65 or over. Married women have the lowest individual incomes of any group regardless of age.

Among the unmarried, there are sex and marital status differences in income (Table 5.1). Among unmarried men under age 65, the divorced have higher incomes ($18,141) than the never married ($13,733), and the widowed ($12,015) have the lowest. For men beyond age 65, the pattern is somewhat different from that of younger men. The widowed have the highest incomes ($7,936) followed by the divorced ($6,991) and never married ($6,833).

Among the younger group of unmarried women, the never married ($12,774) and divorced ($12,652) have substantially higher incomes than the widowed ($9,134). In old age, never-married women have higher incomes ($8,654) than the divorced ($6,777) and widowed ($6,568) women. The only group in which the income of unmarried women exceeds that of unmarried men is among the never married aged 65 and over.

Clearly, the lower incomes of the single relative to those of married couples persist into later life and, of course, have implications for postretirement income. In preretirement years (ages 55 to 65), for example, the relative difference in median income of older married and single men is marked; married men have median incomes that are 78 percent higher than those of their single peers. The relative difference in median income, however, narrows at older ages. Even so, at age 73 married men still have median incomes that are 24 percent greater than those of unmarried men (Marsh, 1981). Bernard concluded that "Marriage is an asset in a man's career, including his earning power" (Bernard, 1972). The effect of marital status on earnings is maintained despite educational levels; single college graduates, for example, have about the same income as married high school graduates (Spreitzer & Riley, 1974).

One way to view the comparative financial situation of the unmarried is to see what proportion are living below an arbitrary poverty threshold. The poverty rate among the aged declined from 35.2 in 1959 to 12.4 percent in 1984 (U.S. Bureau of the Census, 1986). Despite the improved financial conditions of the aged as a group, substrata of the elderly still confront severe economic hardships. Poverty is most acute for the very old, minorities, and aged women who live alone (Warlick, 1985). More elderly females are in poverty (15 percent) than elderly males (8.7 percent). Race is also an important factor. At the same time that poverty among the aged has declined, differences between the races have widened (U.S. Bureau of the Census, 1986).

In 1984, the poverty rate among black elderly was 31.7 percent. Gender differences also persist across races with more black female elderly in poverty (35.5) than black males (26.0). Gender differences combine with marital status so that when older unmarried women are considered as a group, they are most disadvantaged. They more often have postretirement incomes below the poverty level than do unmarried men or couples (Friedman & Sjogren, 1981). Among older female households, the highest probability of being in poverty was found among the separated/divorced, followed by the widowed and never married. Never-married females, however, are relatively well-off compared to other females in terms of an income to needs ratio (Iijima, 1987).

The net worth of the unmarried in retirement is substantially below that of the married (Friedman & Sjogren, 1981). As a whole, with regard to both net worth as well as income, unmarried women begin retirement in an especially difficult economic position. Moreover, assets of unmarried women are more likely to be held in equity in a home than are those of married or unmarried men. A need for liquid assets would probably represent a greater threat to the independence of unmarried women than to that of unmarried men or married couples.

The differential incomes of married and single persons may reflect earlier social and economic discrimination against the unmarried (Stein, 1976). Singles of both sexes experience discrimination in work (hiring, promotion, salary), credit, insurance, and housing (Stein, 1976). Clearly, lifelong discrimination results in reduced income as well as diminished benefits at retirement and possibly lower levels of savings.

How persons come to be unmarried in old age obviously varies, and this may have consequences for financial well-being. Of course, one of the distinguishing characteristics between the never married and formerly married is the change in status experienced by the latter group. But the losses sustained by the divorced and widowed occur under different circumstances, and their consequences may differ for men and women. Whereas both widowers and widows, for example, will have adjusted to bereavement and the social-psychological outcomes of loss of a spouse, Morgan (1981) observed that the objective consequences generally are believed to differ for men and women.

One of the most pervasive objective consequences of both widowhood (Hess & Waring, 1983) and divorce, especially for women, is the loss of income and the subsequent change in financial circumstances (DeShane & Brown-Wilson, 1981). Hess and Waring (1983) concluded that the status of older divorced women is precarious compared to that of their widowed age peers. They posited that earlier disadvantages surrounding the economic impact of divorce culminate in old age to reduce the capacity of these women for autonomy and self-sufficiency.

Uhlenberg and Myers (1981:279) observed that financial security of the aged is "often precariously based upon ownership of house and basic consumer durables." In divorce settlements property may be divided resulting in diminished economic circumstances for both former spouses. Whereas the financial outcomes of being unmarried may be differentiated to an extent by sex, there may be differences by marital status within sex categories as well. For example, in most instances, widowed men are less likely to experience substantially reduced finances, whereas divorced men may sustain a decline in both income and assets.

Subjective Evaluations of Finances and Marital Status

Beyond its consequences for objective income and assets, marital status may also influence subjective evaluations of various domains of life. Compiling data from several national samples, Uhlenberg and Myers (1981) showed that financial satisfaction differed little between older widowed and never-married persons. And there was little variation by sex in evaluations of financial circumstances for the widowed and never married. The divorced/separated, however, were considerably more dissatisfied than other unmarried persons, and older divorced men were most distressed about their financial situation (Uhlenberg & Myers, 1981). Campbell et al. (1976:421) also found that the situation of the divorced was more stressful than that of persons in other marital statuses, and they described the lives of divorced women as "unrelievedly negative." The divorced were the most negative of all women in many domains of life, but they were especially troubled by their standard of living and savings. Campbell et al. found marked differences between divorced men and women, but they were the reverse of those reported by Uhlenberg and Myers. For example, 58 percent of the divorced men never worried about meeting expenses compared to 30 percent of the women (Campbell et al., 1976). However, analyses showing divorced men less satisfied than women with their economic circumstances (Uhlenberg & Myers, 1981; Hyman, 1983) were based on older samples, whereas Campbell's divorced sample included all ages.

Limited available research on older divorced persons suggests then that divorced men may be more burdened by unfavorable evaluations of their finances than are divorced women although the objective financial situation of men is usually more favorable. It may be that the greater strains found among divorced women in multiage samples reflect, in part, the stresses and financial responsibilities for children so that in later life when children are gone, the subjective financial status of women is improved. But the tentative nature of these findings on subjective evaluations of finances should be noted. Even by combining respondents in national surveys conducted from 1972 to 1978, for example, data were obtained for only 46 older divorced/separated men and 76 women (Hyman, 1983). Nevertheless, available research is informative in identifying general differences among the widowed, divorced/separated, and never married in old age. Based on previous research and the potential for earlier economic losses to have cumulative effects in old age, it was expected that the divorced would fare less well on objective income, experience greater financial hardship, compare themselves more negatively with others, and have less satisfaction with their level of living than the never married or widowed.

Factors Associated with Satisfaction with Level of Living

A portion of a model proposed by Campbell et al. (1976) and investigated previously with community samples (Liang, Kahana, & Doherty, 1980) and older married men (Keith, 1985) guided the examination of factors that were linked to satisfaction. The model posits that the influence of background and/or objective characteristics on satisfaction with a specific domain of life is mediated by subjective assessments. Two types of subjective assessments that may intervene between background characteristics and/or objective indices of life domains and satisfaction with a domain were considered in this chapter. One of these was the subjective assessment of the current situation in the domain of finances; in this analysis, evaluation of current financial circumstances was represented by perceptions of financial hardship. A second process that may mediate between objective characteristics and domain satisfaction is the evaluation of one's own situation relative to that of others. In this research the unmarried compared their level of living with that of others. Outcomes of these comparisons may reflect deprivation or disadvantage. Feelings of deprivation or disadvantage are then relative and not absolute (Crosby, 1982). Presumably, satisfaction with a domain involves a complex process that depends, in part, on implicit or explicit social comparisons. It was expected that feelings of satisfaction or dissatisfaction with level of living would derive from both assessments of financial adequacy and relative deprivation based on social comparisons.

Although in research on older married men it was found that income had a direct effect on general life satisfaction (Keith, 1985), most studies suggest that objective indices have an indirect effect on satisfaction with a domain (Campbell et al., 1976; Liang, Kahana, & Doherty, 1980). Therefore, it was anticipated that income would be associated with assessments of financial hardship and would figure in calculations of relative deprivation, but that income would not have a direct influence on satisfaction with level of living.

PROCEDURES

Financial hardship was assessed by the question: "Which of the following four statements describes your ability to get along on your income? I can't make ends meet (1); I have just enough, no more (2); I have enough, with a little extra sometimes (3); I always have money left over (4)."

Satisfaction with level of living was measured by the question: "Generally, how satisfied are you with the way you are living now—that is, as far as money and what you are able to have are concerned? Would you say the way you are living is very unsatisfactory (1) to more than satisfactory (4)." Comparison of level of living with that of others was assessed by asking "Would you say the way you are living is worse than (1), about the same as (2), or better than (3) that of most of your friends and acquaintances?" Data were obtained on the finance measures at both interviews. Higher scores on financial adequacy, satisfaction, and comparisons indicated more positive assessments.

Analyses

Hierarchical multiple regression analyses of satisfaction with level of living and financial hardship were conducted for formerly married and never-married men and women separately. In the first model, satisfaction with level of living at time 1 was examined in relation to satisfaction at time 2. In a second model the effects of age, race, education, income, employment status, health, comparisons of finances, financial hardship, and marital status (for the formerly married) were net of the effects of satisfaction with level of living at time 1. In a third model, race X income and race X marital status effects were included controlling for satisfaction with level of living at time 1 and the background variables used in the second model. Models evaluated for financial hardship were comparable. T-tests and one-way analyses of variance were used to examine differences in satisfaction and hardship by sex and marital status.

RESULTS

Sex and Evaluation of Finances

Assessment of satisfaction with level of living, comparisons of finances with those of others, and financial hardship were largely undifferentiated by sex for the sample as a whole. At the beginning of the decade, men maintained more favorable comparisons of their financial situation than women ($t = 2.03$, $p < .05$), and they less often endured financial hardship ($t = 4.15$, $p < .001$). Later in their lives, however, satisfaction, comparisons, and hardship experienced by men and women were comparable ($t = 1.51$; 1.01; 1.26 respectively).

Sex and Income of the Unmarried

In Chapter 2, it was reported that men had significantly higher incomes than women at both time 1 and time 2. This, of course, is a conventional finding in the literature for preretirement income, and it is generally thought that the discrepancy would extend beyond the working years. Sex differences in income were not found for the divorced and never married ($t = .77$; $.85$, ns, respectively); however, widowed men enjoyed substantially higher incomes than widows ($t = 2.45$, $p < .05$). In the next sections, I consider differences by marital status for women and men.

Marital Status and Finances of Women

Separate one-way analyses of variance of marital status and assessments of finances were conducted for women and men. The three evaluations of finances (satisfaction with level of living; financial hardship; and comparisons) at both time 1 and time 2 provided six tests of the effect of marital status for men and women and supplied evidence on the relationship between marital status and finances at the beginning and end of a decade.

Marital status differentiated the financial circumstances of women more often than those of men; on each of the six tests marital status of women was linked with subjective assessments of finances. At both interviews, marital status was significantly associated with satisfaction with level of living ($F = 17.50$, $p < .001$; $F = 14.22$, $p < .001$), financial hardship ($F = 20.74$, $p < .001$; $F = 19.75$, $p < .001$), and comparisons of level of living with that of others ($F = 3.29$, $p < .05$; $F = 5.98$, $p < .01$).

At both the beginning and end of the decade divorced women gave significantly more negative assessments of their financial condition than the never married. In all instances but one, the widowed also were less positive than the never married about their circumstances. Furthermore, although the divorced were most negative about their situation, the widowed usually did not hold significantly more positive attitudes than the divorced. By the end of the decade, widowed and divorced women held comparable views of their financial circumstances (on all three measures) that were substantially more negative than those of the never married. Moreover, at both interviews subjective assessments corresponded to the relationship between actual income and marital status. Widowed and divorced women had significantly lower incomes than the never married at time 1 ($F = 15.78$, $p < .001$) and at time 2 ($F = 19.23$, $p < .001$). Furthermore, the subjective assessments also may have reflected the increments in income over the decade since never-married women had the largest increases followed by widowed and divorced women.

Marital Status and Finances of Men

Marital status of men was linked with assessments of financial conditions on three of the six subjective measures. Marital status was associated with comparisons with others at time 1 ($F = 8.60$, $p < .001$) and at time 2 with satisfaction with level of living ($F = 6.01$, $p < .01$) and financial hardship ($F = 13.75$, $p < .001$). Thus marital status differentiated the financial concerns of men less than those of women. When marital status was a factor in assessments of financial circumstances, however, the divorced were always more negative than the widowed and never married. In contrast to divorced and widowed women, who viewed their circumstances similarly, among men the widowed were more like the never married suggesting that their lives may have had less financial disruption.

Differences in income by marital status followed a comparable pattern to that of subjective assessments in which marital status influenced income at the end of the decade ($F = 7.18$, $p < .001$) but not at time 1. At the end of the ten-year period, divorced men had significantly lower incomes than the never married with the widowed occupying an intermediate position. Moreover, divorced men had the smallest increments in income over the decade of any sex or marital status group. Thus over time marital status came to have a closer link to both subjective evaluations of finances and income of men than earlier.

Dissatisfaction, Hardship, and Comparative Deprivation

To indicate the extent to which these unmarried experienced difficulties and to describe those with the most marked problems, Table 5.2 shows percentages of persons by sex and marital status who found their level of living very unsatisfactory, felt financially deprived relative to others, and who could not get along on their income. Ten percent or fewer of all groups of the unmarried found their level of living very unsatisfactory. The never married were least likely (less than 5 percent) to evaluate their level of living as very unsatisfactory.

About one-quarter or more of the divorced men and women believed their level of living compared unfavorably with that of their age peers. Over the decade as a group, the proportions of divorced who experienced comparative deprivation declined slightly (from 28 to 24 percent for men and 29 to 24 percent for women) but about one-fourth still felt they were worse off than others. Among the widowed and never married, women were a little more likely than men to draw unfavorable comparisons both earlier and later in their lives.

Investigation of extreme financial hardship, at the beginning and end of the decade, indicated that widowed men and never-married men and women experienced the least hardship and divorced men and women the most. For example, more than one-quarter of these divorced men continued to have financial hardship so severe that they could not get along on their incomes at the end of the decade.

Table 5.2
Dissatisfaction, Negative Comparisons, and Financial Hardship
by Sex and Marital Status (Percentages)

	Men					
	Widowed		Divorced		Never Married	
	Time 1	Time 2	Time 1	Time 2	Time 1	Time 2
Very Unsatisfactory Level of Living	9	7	12	11	3	4
Negative Comparisons with Others	17	16	28	24	14	14
Financial Hardship	18	14	29	27	7	10

	Women					
	Widowed		Divorced		Never Married	
	Time 1	Time 2	Time 1	Time 2	Time 1	Time 2
Very Unsatisfactory Level of Living	7	7	11	10	3	4
Negative Comparisons with Others	22	20	29	24	19	15
Financial Hardship	23	19	28	22	15	13

Fewer of the widowed and never-married men experienced inadequate incomes during the same time.

Multivariate Analyses of Satisfaction with Level of Living

Three models of satisfaction with level of living were considered in hierarchical regression analyses for formerly married men and women and never-married men and women. In the first model, satisfaction with level of living at time 1 was investigated in relation to later satisfaction (Table 5.3). In addition to satisfaction at time 1, the second model included age, race, income, education, employment status, health, financial hardship, comparison of finances, and marital status (for the formerly married). A third model was comprised of race X income and race X marital status effects as well as the variables included in models one and two.

Table 5.3
Regression Analyses of Satisfaction with Level of Living by Sex and Marital Status

| | Widowed/Divorced | | | | | | | | Never Married | | | | | | |
| | Males | | | | Females | | | | Males | | | Females | | | |
	r	Model I Beta	Model II Beta	Model III Beta	r	Model I Beta	Model II Beta	Model III Beta	r	Model I Beta	Model II Beta	r	Model I Beta	Model II Beta	Model III Beta
Satisfaction with level living (Time 1)	.39	.39**	.25**	.24**	.33	.33**	.18**	.18**	.17	.17**	.06	.26	.26**	.07	.07
Age	.04	—	-.05	-.06	.01	—	.01	.01	-.09	—	-.03	.02	—	.00	.01
Race	-.03	—	.02	.21	-.09	—	.01	.14**	—	—	—	-.16	—	-.04*	.01
Income	.26	—	-.01	.05	.28	—	.05*	.06	.28	—	.06	.30	—	.06	.06
Education	.00	—	-.07	-.08	.13	—	-.06**	.06	.06	—	.00	.18	—	-.04	-.05
Employment status	.06	—	-.01	-.00	.14	—	.03	-.06**	.11	—	.03	-.01	—	-.04	-.03
Health	.19	—	.06	.06	.22	—	.07**	.07**	.25	—	.16**	.16	—	.06	.06
Financial hardship	.45	—	.31**	.31**	.48	—	.34**	.34**	.38	—	.22**	.51	—	.35**	.34**
Comparison of finances	.33	—	.19**	.19**	.37	—	.22**	.22**	.40	—	.26**	.45	—	.31**	.31
Marital status	-.13	—	-.04	-.03	-.04	—	-.00	-.00	—	—	—	—	—	—	—
Race x Income	-.03	—	—	-.23*	-.07	—	—	-.14**	—	—	—	-.15	—	—	-.06*
Race x Marital status	-.05	—	—	.02	-.03	—	—	-.01	—	—	—	—	—	—	—
Change in R^2	—	—	.161	.011	—	—	.219	.003	—	—	.227	—	—	.295	.001
R^2	—	.149	.310	.321	—	.112	.331	.334	—	.028	.255	—	.067	.362	.363

* $p < .10$
** $p < .05$

As expected, in the initial model, assessments of level of living at time 1 had significant effects on satisfaction with level of living later in the decade for men and women regardless of marital status. Early evaluations of satisfaction, however, were less salient among never-married men and women and explained only three and seven percent of the variance in their later assessments compared to eleven and fifteen percent for formerly married women and men. Moreover, the influence of satisfaction at time 1 remained strong when additional variables were considered for the formerly married. The weaker relationship between assessments of satisfaction with level of living over time for the never married suggests less stability in satisfaction for them.

In the second model, background characteristics (e.g., age, race, education) and assessments of financial hardship and comparisons with others were included along with the time 1 measure of satisfaction. (Because of the small number of minority men, race was excluded from the model for never-married men.) Background characteristics, financial hardship, and comparisons were important in explaining satisfaction and accounted for 16 percent of the variance among formerly married men and ranged to 29 percent among never-married women (Table 5.3). Marital status (widowed vs. divorced) did not differentiate satisfaction with level of living of the formerly married. Rather, perceptions of financial hardship and feelings of comparative deprivation were important in fostering dissatisfaction with level of living. The bivariate relationship between health and satisfaction with level of living was positive for all groups although when other characteristics were considered, poor health was a minor factor in dissatisfaction for most. In the second model, satisfaction at time 1 was no longer important in explaining satisfaction at the end of the decade for never-married men and women.

Higher income was correlated with satisfaction with level of living. For the most part in the final model, income did not have a direct effect on views of level of living, and the effect of income on satisfaction was mediated through assessments of financial hardship. Relationships between income and assessments of financial hardship ranged from $r = .45$ to .60. In contrast, perceptions of relative deprivation as revealed in comparisons of one's own finances with those of others were largely independent of actual income especially among widowed men ($r = .04$) and women ($r = .13$), divorced women ($r = -.01$), and never-married women ($r = .08$). Income figured more prominently in feelings of deprivation of divorced ($r = .30$) and never-married men (r = .26). Even so, the effect of income on satisfaction with level of living was mediated through perceptions of financial hardship rather than relative deprivation for the majority.

In the final model, there were significant race × income interaction effects for satisfaction with level of living among formerly married men and women (Table 5.3). Further analyses indicated that among low-income formerly married men and women, satisfaction with level of living was not differentiated by race. Rather, black men ($\bar{X}$ = 2.62) and women (2.60) with higher incomes indicated less satisfaction than white men ($\bar{X}$ = 2.85) and women ($\bar{X}$ = 2.92) with comparable earnings.

The full model explained comparable amounts of variance in satisfaction with level of living among women regardless of marital status (over 30 percent for each group) and formerly married men (32 percent). The predictors were less efficient for never-married men, accounting for about 25 percent of the variance in satisfaction with level of living. However, factors that were most salient to satisfaction with level of living were fairly comparable across sex and marital status groups.

Additional regression analyses for satisfaction with level of living that are not reported in detail here were conducted for the widowed and divorced separately. Employment at the end of the decade was associated with satisfaction with level of living only among divorced women (r = .24), but it had little effect on the satisfaction of any other group. Generally, in the separate analyses by marital status, however, background characteristics (e.g., age, race, education) continued to have a less direct effect on satisfaction with level of living than subjective assessments (i.e., time 1 attitudes, comparisons with others, or evaluations of financial hardship).

Multivariate Analyses of Financial Hardship

Three models similar to those for satisfaction with level of living were investigated for financial hardship. In the first model, the influence of early financial hardship at time 1 on later assessments was examined. In the second model, in addition to hardship at time 1, other demographic and attitudinal variables were included (age, race, income, education, employment status, health, comparison of finances, and marital status (for the formerly married)). The third model was comprised of two interaction effects (race × income and race × marital status) as well as the variables included in the previous two models.

In the initial model, assessments of hardship at time 1 had a significant effect on financial difficulties experienced later in life regardless of gender or marital status. But the effect was considerably stronger for some than others (Table 5.4). Perceptions of hardship by never-married men at the end of the decade, for example, were least influenced by earlier financial problems. Initial evaluations of never-married men explained only 9 percent of the variance in later hardship compared to 27 percent for never-married women.

In the second model, background characteristics (e.g., age, race, education, income, health) and comparisons with others were included along with the time 1 measure of hardship. After the effect of hardship at time 1 was removed, background characteristics and comparisons accounted for 17 percent of the variance in financial hardship for the formerly married, 23 percent for never-married women, and 26 percent for never-married men. Higher income directly diminished hardship regardless of marital status and gender. At the same time, negative comparative assessments of their financial situation also contributed to perceptions of greater hardship for all groups.

In the final model, there was a significant race by marital status interaction effect for financial hardship among formerly married men. Additional analyses indicated that there were no differences between black and white widowers in their experience of financial hardship ($\bar{X} = 2.36$, 2.39, respectively) whereas divorced black men reported more difficulties with income adequacy ($\bar{X} = 1.94$) than their white counterparts ($\bar{X} = 2.13$). Further examination of the significant race by income effect for never-married women revealed that high income did not mitigate perceptions of hardship among black women. Indeed, high-income black women viewed their financial situation as more precarious and difficult ($\bar{X} = 2.00$) than even low-income white women ($\bar{X} = 2.20$). In contrast, white women with high incomes saw their lives as substantially freer of hardship ($\bar{X} = 3.21$) although it must be observed that low-income black women faced the most hardship of any group of never-married women ($\bar{X} = 1.72$).

Separate regression analyses for widowed and divorced women indicated the importance of continued employment for both in reducing financial hardship although involvement in the labor force especially diminished perceptions of financial inadequacy among divorced women. Moreover, the income of divorced women was more contingent on employment ($r = .32$) than that of any other group. For most, the relationship between work and income was more modest; for example, $r = .05$ and .19 for never-married women and widows, respectively.

Healthier widowed and divorced women also experienced less hardship, but those in better health were also more often employed (r = .20, .30, respectively). Age was a positive factor for divorced women since they experienced somewhat less hardship if they were older (r = .10; B = .15) whereas education seemed to offset financial inadequacy especially for widowed women (r = .31; B = .06).

SUMMARY AND DISCUSSION

This chapter has provided observations about the financial situation of the unmarried both earlier and later in their lives. Marital status differentiated the perceptions of finances and economic circumstances of men somewhat less than those of women. Even so, among men, the divorced were most disadvantaged in level of income, increments in income over the ten-year period, and in subjective assessments of finances at the close of the decade. The financial situation and perceptions of widowed men more closely resembled those of the never married suggesting that loss of a spouse alone was not the critical factor in determining views of financial circumstances. Because divorced men were relatively more deprived than other unmarried men at the end of decade, divorce may have had a cumulative negative effect on these older men.

In contrast to the situation for men, divorced and widowed women tended to have similar financial circumstances and were more disadvantaged than the never married on both subjective measures and in income at both interviews. Thus these data did not corroborate the conclusion of Hyman (1983:81) that widowed women had "fortified their spirits against severe deprivation" and reported satisfaction with their finances that was unwarranted by their actual situation. In the present research, widows' assessments of how well they were faring reflected their more limited financial resources over time. Neither did they aggrandize their financial circumstances relative to the appraisals of men.

Of course, the greater hardship of the widowed and divorced women compared with the never married may have been antecedent to the dissolution of their marriages and have characterized their lives in years prior to the study (Morgan, 1981), although data were not available to test this. Formerly married women may have been more disadvantaged over the decade than never-married women, in part, due to their employment in lower level occupations. At the beginning of the decade never-married women were employed in significantly higher level occupations than formerly married women, and they also may have had more sustained career histories. Therefore, the data suggested that observations on the precariousness of the situation of divorced women (Hess & Waring, 1983) could be extended to the financial domain of these widowed women and to a lesser extent to divorced men.

In general, the models that explained satisfaction with level of living were relatively similar for the various sex and marital status groups. None of the background characteristics had a consistent and significant direct effect on satisfaction across all of the groups. In contrast to demographic characteristics, assessments of financial hardship were salient in satisfaction with level of living regardless of sex or marital status. Age peers provided a frame of reference for self-assessments so that evaluations resulting from the comparisons were important in determining attitudes toward level of living. Those who appraised their financial situation as more advantaged relative to others were more contented with their level of living.

Campbell et al. (1976) found that the association between income as an objective resource and subjective reports of satisfaction with financial situations was weaker than the fit between objective indices and satisfaction with other resource domains such as friendships and health. In the present research, income for various groups was correlated with satisfaction with level of living (r = .26 to .30), but when other variables were controlled, income did not have a direct effect on satisfaction. It might be assumed that level of income would figure into the calculations of how well persons felt they were living relative to their acquaintances. Relative deprivation, however, tended to be independent of money for most of the sample, that is, for all women and widowed men. Income though influenced perceptions of adequacy of income (i.e., whether persons were unable to make ends meet or had some left over) that in turn affected satisfaction.

Perhaps reflecting their greater financial needs, both divorced women and men tended to have somewhat higher rates of employment than most of their counterparts at the end of the decade. Divorced women had the highest rate of employment at time 2, 18 percent, followed by divorced and never-married men with 16 percent at work compared with 10 to 12 percent for widowed men and women and never-married women. Separate analyses for widowed and divorced women indicating the salience of employment to satisfaction with level of living only among the divorced may have underscored their financial deprivation. Even with higher rates of employment their incomes tended to be lower than those of any other sex and marital status group.

When race did impact views of finances, it was most often in conjunction with some other dimension for example, marital status or income. Furthermore, the lack of correspondence between the objective income of blacks and their subjective assessments of their financial situation was particularly salient. Especially those with higher incomes did not have the accompanying psychic benefits of satisfaction with their attainments or relief from hardship and difficulty in making ends meet. It may be that the demands on unmarried blacks with a higher income are overwhelming and burdensome belying what is often viewed as a single status unencumbered by the financial obligations of a family. Blacks may provide and be expected to extend more support and help to their families (Brubaker, 1985). The burden may be especially heavy for the higher income unmarried individual and perhaps more so for women than for men. Although literature suggests that sons, more than daughters, provide economic help to parents in old age, it is possible that unmarried men and women may be seen as having fewer demands on their income and more available to share and distribute to others. It may be that such a situation leaves some unable to meet their own needs. Furthermore, unmarried women may be especially targeted for demands; women may be regarded as more empathetic and approachable. Another explanation for the seeming discrepancy between objective income and subjective observations about their economic situation by higher income unmarried blacks might be that the success they were able to attain reflected in better incomes fell short of their rising expectations.

This chapter has considered the consequences of nonmarriage in old age for the financial domain of life. There was evidence that the strains of divorce and widowhood for women and divorce for older men had an enduring influence on finances and in the instance of men these concerns were heightened over the ten-year period. It has been observed that marriage does not preclude economic difficulties, rather it aids persons in avoiding some of the psychological problems that might otherwise emanate from such events (Pearlin & Johnson, 1977). Among the unmarried in this sample, especially for women and to a lesser degree men, not ever having married seemed to perform a similar function with respect to responses to economic difficulties in old age. Earlier decisions for careers in higher level occupations and more sustained participation in the work force by never-married women were rewarded by more positive assessments of finances in later life and more appreciative evaluations of their circumstances.

Work, Retirement, and Well-Being   **6**

One objective of this chapter is to investigate whether the unmarried differed in their assessments of work, retirement, and well-being. A further interest is in the examination of factors associated with evaluations of work, retirement, and global happiness among these widowed, divorced/separated, and never-married older men and women. It has been suggested that work may be especially important to the unmarried since it is a form of involvement that may compensate for the absence of gratification derived from marriage (Ward, 1979). Furthermore, if work represents such an important tie to the community and provides opportunities for social contacts, then withdrawal from work may result in diminished well-being for the unmarried. Examination of these issues may be of use to practitioners and preretirement planners. Szinovacz (1983) emphasized the need to investigate factors that affect retirement adjustment in divergent population groups indicating such research may provide a basis for intervention. Beck (1982) has also called for research to specify further the groups or types of retirees that may have difficulty in adjusting to retirement.

WORK AND THE UNMARRIED

It has been observed that despite discrimination in the work place, singles report high commitment to work; for example, among single adults, work and a fulfilling career were among the most important goals in life (Braito & Anderson, 1983). Using a national survey as their base, Veroff et al. (1981) concluded that single men and women derived more of their social validity from work than did their married peers and that "They are especially sensitive to their reputation as workers." In a study of women, Birnbaum (1975) observed that work serves as a "major source of self-worth and financial and emotional security for the never-married professional."

There is some evidence that evaluations of work may vary by sex among the unmarried (Veroff et al., 1981). Veroff et al. (1981) found that work was more critical to older unmarried women than to older unmarried men. Both previously married and never-married women found greater value fulfillment through work than did their male counterparts. These findings for the unmarried represent a departure from literature that suggests work is less salient in the lives of women than in those of men and, hence, attachment to work would have less impact on the retirement adjustment of the former (Matthews & Brown, 1987). Whereas single men were more likely than married men to emphasize fulfillment of values through leisure compared to work, the opposite was true for women. Even so, both unmarried men and women found validation through work to a greater extent than did married persons.

But marital status as a major organizing status throughout life may have different implications for work orientations within the unmarried groups especially for women. Married and formerly married women likely will have had shorter work careers than men or never-married women. Married and formerly married women may hold numerous jobs with little or no advancement as they move in and out of the labor force. The qualitative character of married women's job histories seem to be shaped by their family roles, their socialization to work and the workplace, and the historical period (Keating & Jeffrey, 1983). It has been assumed that never-married women have had less interrupted work careers, in part, because of their need to support themselves and because they devote time to work instead of family responsibilities (Keating & Jeffrey, 1983).

If family obligations influence the work roles of married women in ways that they do not intrude on the career experiences of men and never-married women, then we might expect that attitudes of never-married women would be differentiated from those of formerly married women. Because of presumed conflicts between worker and spouse roles, Atchley (1976) posited that women who were married or who had been married would have a less positive orientation to work. When income was controlled, he found the never-married women had a stronger work orientation than the formerly married.

In other research it was found that about twice as many never-married women (32 percent) as previously married women (17 percent) believed they received more social validation through their work than they would have through marriage or parenthood (Veroff et al., 1981). There was a comparable pattern of validation from work for men by marital status although there was less difference between the never married (28 percent) and previously married (23 percent).

RETIREMENT AND THE UNMARRIED

If work is highly salient to the unmarried, this raises the question of how they manage the loss of work and whether retirement has a differential impact on the formerly married and never married. In general, there has been little support for the view that retirement is a predominantly negative experience characterized by great loss and crisis (Foner & Schwab, 1981; Mutran & Reitzes, 1981). Rather, most are satisfied with retirement, do not experience deteriorating health as a consequence, and do not want to resume work. Although retirement has beneficial as well as negative outcomes, the detrimental consequences are small or insignificant (Palmore, Fillenbaum, & George, 1984).

Ward (1979), however, observed that retirement had a more negative effect on the happiness of the never married than of the married. Using happiness as one indicator, Ward concluded that the loss of work was more consequential for the never married since they lacked structured family roles. Many of the formerly married, of course, at some time may have had such family roles. Comparisons of the effects of retirement on happiness of the widowed and divorced/separated were not presented. Thus, available information on attitudes toward retirement by the unmarried is too limited to state specific hypotheses about different patterns by marital status.

GENDER AND ADJUSTMENT TO RETIREMENT

A further question is whether there are sex differences among the unmarried in their adjustment to retirement. Some research suggests a possible link between older women's work orientation and adaptation to retirement. Work orientations of older females may be differentiated from those of males because "Career-oriented women must focus their resources and energies to a greater extent than career-oriented men to overcome financial, social, and psychological obstacles to careers for women" (Ward, 1979). Because this heightened commitment may deflect women from marriage, it may also influence the difficulty with which they withdraw from work. Of course, educational attainment and occupational levels may figure in the attachment to work and retirement as well. Although Ward found that the never married had more difficulty with retirement than the married, he did not control for sex.

A contrasting approach projects a different view of work orientation and a different response to retirement by suggesting that the majority of the present generation of older women anticipated that work would be secondary to family obligations and that leaving work would be easy since it meant returning to the familiar setting of the home. Implicit in this perspective is that: (a) women have a low commitment to work; (b) their central role is located outside the workplace; (c) they have an acceptable role to resume and can do so with few changes; (d) work makes a minimal contribution to their self esteem; (e) and, hence, it has little effect on their life satisfaction or subsequent adjustment in retirement (Gratton & Haug, 1983; Keating & Jeffrey, 1983). The argument that work is less important to women and, therefore, retirement will be easier for them, overlooks those for whom family may not be a primary role, for example, never-married women with a sustained career pattern and commitment to an occupation, women who are single heads of households, and men who attach greater importance to family or other life areas than to work (Gee & Kimball, 1987).

In contrast to the view that retirement will involve a smooth transition, some research has suggested that women have more problems than men in adjusting to retirement (Atchley, 1976; Palmore, 1984; Szinovacz, 1982). Recently Seccombe and Lee (1986) reported that women had lower levels of retirement satisfaction than men although the differences, while statistically significant, were small. In comparison with men, greater difficulties experienced by women have been reflected in things they miss in retirement—the feeling of doing a good job, social contacts and also loneliness, less satisfaction with retirement, and financial strain. Levy (1980) found that negative retirement attitudes have more prolonged effects on the adjustment of women than of men. Gratton and Haug (1983), however, criticized much of the research for its specific occupational samples, single sex samples, and/or small samples.

In the present research the influence of background characteristics (e.g., age, education, occupation), health, income, and employment status were considered in relation to attitudes toward work, retirement, and happiness. Health consistently has been found to be a primary factor in determining satisfaction with life (Elwell & Maltbie-Crannell, 1981) and with retirement (Foner & Schwab, 1981; Seccombe & Lee, 1986). Persons in poor health hold more negative attitudes toward retirement and moreover they have a greater number of problems that continue into retirement (Atchley & Robinson, 1982). There is evidence that health may affect assessments of retirement somewhat differently for men and women. Atchley (1982) concluded that the adverse effects of poor health figured more importantly in depressing the retirement attitudes of women than of men. Early retirement is often prompted by poor health, but there is little evidence that retirement itself fosters deterioration in health (Palmore et al., 1984).

Generally research has found a positive relationship between income and men's attitudes toward retirement (Barfield & Morgan, 1978; Beck, 1982; Foner & Schwab, 1981; Hatch, 1987). Men with lower incomes feel more negative toward retirement both before and after they leave employment. As in the instance of health, women with inadequate incomes hold more negative attitudes than men in comparable financial straits (Atchley, 1982). Assurance of a higher income in retirement seems to prompt early retirement.

The association between occupational level and attitudes toward retirement is quite unclear since research shows inverse, curvilinear, and positive relationships (see Hatch, 1987, for a review). Occupations may differentially prepare individuals for retirement although some research indicates the relationship between occupational level and attitudes toward retirement diminishes or disappears when health and income are controlled (Seccomb & Lee, 1986). Rather, better health and higher income may enhance satisfaction with retirement more directly than any skills or preparation for retirement that may have been derived from occupational placement. Education has also been found to be related to satisfaction with life in general and with retirement (Campbell, Converse, & Rodgers, 1976). Ward (1979) concluded that education in addition to health and income was a better predictor of happiness of the never-married aged than of the married. Because these resources are important to the aged regardless of marital status, they may be especially salient in the absence of a spouse. Earlier, I referred to the observation of Stein (1976) that singleness is hard, but resources of health, income, and education may help foster physical mobility, cultivation of a variety of interests, and flexibility needed to maintain a more independent lifestyle. Presumably these resources would be reflected in evaluations of retirement and happiness.

Finally, morale or satisfaction in retirement may be due to aspects of life other than ceasing work per se (Seccombe & Lee, 1986). Financial or health problems, for example, rather than the absence of work itself, may foster low morale or dissatisfaction in retirement (Foner & Schwab, 1981; Riddick, 1985). In this chapter, evaluations of work, retirement, and happiness of the unmarried are considered in relation to sex, age, race, education, occupation, income, health, and employment status.

PROCEDURES: MEASURES

Attitudes toward Work

Attitudes toward work were assessed by summing responses to two items: "Work is the most meaningful part of life" and "Most people think more of someone who works than they do of someone who doesn't." Response categories ranged from "Strongly agree" (4) to "Strongly disagree" (1) with a high score indicating a more positive orientation toward work.

Attitudes toward Retirement

Attitudes toward retirement were assessed by summing responses to three questions: "Retirement is a pleasant time of life"; "People who don't retire when they are financially able are foolish"; "Older workers should retire when they can, so as to give younger people more of a chance of the job." Response categories ranged from "Strongly agree" (4) to "Strongly disagree" (1); a high score represented more positive attitudes toward retirement. These questions were included in the 1971 interview but they are indicated here as time 1 measures since all of them were not asked in 1969.

Happiness

Global happiness was measured by an item frequently used in national surveys: "Taking things altogether, would you say you're very happy (3), pretty happy (2), or not too happy (1) these days?" A higher score indicated greater happiness.

Health

Functional capacity was assessed by summing responses to two questions: "Do you have any health condition, physical handicap, or disability that limits how well you get around?" and "Does your health limit the kind or amount of work or housework you can do?" Response categories "yes" and "no" were coded 0, 1. A higher score indicated greater functional capacity.

Occupation

Occupation was coded into eleven categories ranging from laborer (1) to professional (11). The majority of the men were located in five groups: laborers (10 percent); service workers (12 percent); operatives (21 percent); craftsmen, foremen (16 percent); and managers and proprietors (12 percent). Women were concentrated in the following occupational groups: clerical workers (23 percent); service workers (19 percent); operatives (14 percent); professional, technical (14 percent); and private household workers (13 percent).

Employment status at time 2 was coded 0 (not employed) and 1 (employed). Nineteen percent of the men and 20 percent of the women employed at time 1 were still working at the close of the decade.

Education

Education was grouped in categories ranging from 1 through 6. About one-third (32 percent) of the women and 49 percent of the men had an elementary education or less; 18 percent of the men and 20 percent of the women had some high school; 20 percent of the men and 28 percent of the women were high school graduates; 7 percent of the men and 9 percent of the women had completed college and/or graduate work.

Analyses

Hierarchical multiple regression models of attitudes toward work, retirement, and happiness were considered for the formerly married and never married who were employed at time 1. In the analyses of work and retirement attitudes and happiness, education, occupation, income, and the initial attitude measure were entered as the first block. Employment status, health, and income at time 2 formed the second level in the analyses of attitudes toward work, retirement, and happiness. In the analysis of happiness, evaluations of retirement were included in the second block. Attitudes toward work were excluded from analyses of attitudes toward retirement and happiness because of low correlations between these variables. These analyses were based on the unmarried who were employed in 1969. There were 954 women and 252 men.

RESULTS

Gender and Attitudes toward Work and Retirement

One concern was how attitudes toward work, retirement, and happiness differed by gender within marital status categories. T-tests were used to examine sex differences within each marital status, and one-way analyses of variance were employed to investigate the relationship between marital status and work-retirement attitudes at both time 1 and time 2.

Widowers evaluated work more positively than widows at both the beginning (t = 3.55; p < .001) and end of the decade (t = 2.37; p < .05), and they also held more favorable opinions of retirement (F = 2.01, p < .05; 2.54, p < .05). Divorced men tended to endorse work more than divorced women (F = 2.26, p < .05; 2.16, p < .05). Divorced men were more positive toward retirement than divorced women both earlier and later in their lives (t = 2.75, p < .05; 2.21, p < .005). Never-married men endorsed work more strongly than women at time 1 (F = 2.25, p < .05), but later they shared views of work (F = .16). Earlier their opinions of retirement were similar (t = .19) whereas by the close of the decade women were slightly more favorable to retirement than men (t = 1.87, p < .10). In general, then, widowed and divorced men were more favorably disposed toward both work and retirement than formerly married women whereas never-married men and women tended to be more similar in their views.

Marital Status and Attitudes toward Work and Retirement

Following suggestions in the literature that never-married and formerly married women may regard work and perhaps retirement differently, one-way analyses of variance of marital status and attitudes were performed for women and men separately. Attitudes toward work were not associated with marital status among men ($F = 1.86; 1.71$) or women ($F = 1.33; 1.37$) at either interview.

Widowed men had more positive perceptions of retirement than never-married men by the end of the decade ($F = 3.32$, $p < .05$) although there were no differences by marital status at time 1 ($F = 1.90$). At the beginning of the decade widowed and never-married women had the most positive views of retirement ($F = 2.92$, $p < .05$); never-married women sustained their favorable perceptions of retirement and embraced it more than either widowed or divorced women at the close of the decade ($F = 3.03$, $p < .05$). Attitudes toward work and retirement at time 2 were not related to one another among either men or women ($r = .04; .01$).

Multivariate Analyses of Attitudes toward Work

Table 6.1 shows separate hierarchical regression analyses for evaluations of work at time 2 for formerly married men and women and for the never married. As expected, time 1 attitudes toward work tended to have the strongest effect on later evaluations of work; an exception was for never-married men for whom better health was salient in prompting more favorable attitudes toward work (Table 6.1). For the most part, however, perceptions of work were not related to social status characteristics.

Even inclusion of attitudes toward work at time 1, did not ensure that the models were good predictors of evaluations of work by the unmarried in later life. In general, the models suggested that other aspects of life need to be assessed in relation to attitudes toward work; the explained variance ranged from 10 percent for formerly married women to 17 percent for never-married men (Table 6.1). Earlier analyses indicated that age and race were not significant predictors of attitudes toward work for any of the groups.

Table 6.1
Hierarchical Regression Analyses of Attitudes toward Work and Retirement

	Attitudes toward Work							
	Widowed/Divorced				Never Married			
	Men		Women		Men		Women	
	r	Beta	r	Beta	r	Beta	r	Beta
Attitudes/ Work, Time 1	.30	.30***	.25	.23***	.20	.24***	.32	.31***
Marital Status	.05	.08	.04	.05	--	--	--	--
Education	.01	00	-.18	-.10**	-.09	-.05	.10	.27***
Occupation	.14	.17*	-.16	-.05	.01	.11	-.04	-.22**
R^2	.118		.096		.051		.138	
Health, Time 2	.14	-.08	-.06	-.05	.28	.32***	-.04	-.02
Income	-.01	-.06	-.16	-.06	-.16	-.19*	-.04	-.04
Employment Status	-.04	-.01	.03	.06*	.09	.01	.06	.06
Total R^2	.129		.103		.171		.143	
	Attitudes toward Retirement							
Attitudes/ Retirement, Time 1	.39	.37***	.32	.28***	.35	.30***	.41	.36***
Marital Status	-.02	.02	-.02	.01	--	--	--	--
Education	-.07	.07	-.16	-.09*	-.19	-.08	-.02	-.17
Occupation	-.27	-.13	.12	-.03	-.24	.12	.13	.20**
R^2	.192		.116		.159		.194	
Health, Time 2	.18	.28***	-.03	.04	.17	.13	.16	.15**
Income	-.20	-.15*	-.15	-.04	.01	.07	.04	.01
Employment Status	-.19	-.12	-.18	-.15***	-.16	-.16*	-.23	-.17**
Total R^2	.276		.139		.199		.241	

*p < .10

**p < .05

***p < .01

Multivariate Analyses of Attitudes toward Retirement

Factors that were important determinants of retirement attitudes were comparable, for the most part, across marital statuses (Table 6.1). Generally aspects of socioeconomic position (e.g., income, occupational level) explained little variance in retirement attitudes. Earlier attitudes toward retirement had a significant effect on perceptions regardless of marital status. Positive attitudes toward retirement at the beginning of the decade and withdrawal from the labor force were associated with more positive views toward retirement at time 2 among all persons except formerly married men among whom higher income prompted negative thoughts of retirement. Better health was linked with more favorable assessments of retirement among the formerly married men and never-married women. Never-married women in higher level occupations also tended to view retirement more positively.

The models explained least variance in attitudes toward retirement for formerly married women (14 percent) compared to 28 and 24 percent, respectively, for formerly married men and never-married women (Table 6.1). Finally, earlier analyses (not reported here) indicated that attitudes toward retirement were independent of age and race of these unmarried.

Happiness

At both time 1 and time 2, men and women who were widowed (t = .20; 1.81) or divorced (t = 1.61; 1.67) reported similar levels of happiness, but never-married women enjoyed greater happiness than never-married men both earlier and later in the decade (t = 3.04; p < .01; 2.50, p < .01). In this section a primary interest is in the extent to which attitudes toward retirement were important to happiness when other aspects of life were also considered. That is, were observations about retirement critical to maintaining happiness?

Table 6.2
Hierarchical Regression Analyses of Happiness

	Happiness							
	Widowed/Divorced				Never Married			
	Men		Women		Men		Women	
	r	Beta	r	Beta	r	Beta	r	Beta
Happiness, Time 1	.22	.14*	.38	.30***	.29	.17*	.37	.26***
Marital Status	-.09	-.01	-.03	-.02	--	--	--	--
Education	-.07	-.10	.11	00	-.01	-.02	.23	.08
Occupation	.15	.18*	.18	.10**	-.13	-.12	.27	.09
Age	.18	.11	.06	.06*	-.03	-.02	.03	.02
R^2		.103		.165		.121		.180
Health, Time 2	.32	.25***	.20	.12***	.45	.35***	.26	.16***
Income	.17	.05	.19	.11***	.18	.15	.25	.08
Employment Status	.01	-.01	.09	.05	.08	.07	.11	.11
Attitudes/Retirement	.22	.20**	.20	.21***	.16	.08	.28	.25***
Total R^2		.216		.232		.267		.289

*p < .10

**p < .05

***p < .01

Earlier estimates of happiness contributed significantly to happiness at the later time for all groups studied (Table 6.2). Among single men, however, health had a stronger effect on current happiness than the degree of happiness earlier in the decade. For women regardless of marital status, health was less important to happiness than attitudes toward retirement.

Employment status per se was not an important factor, but evaluations of retirement were very salient for all groups except never-married men for whom health had an especially strong effect on happiness. Illustrating their salience, retirement attitudes were either more important or of similar significance as happiness at time 1 in predicting happiness enjoyed by formerly married men and never-married women at the end of the decade. This suggests that happiness was not very stable over the decade, and current feelings about retirement overshadowed earlier assessments of well-being.

Projected Financial Problems in Retirement

At time 1, respondents not yet retired indicated whether retirement would bring financial problems for them. Forty-five percent of those responding (n = 689) observed that retirement would be accompanied by financial problems for them. There was a tendency for women to anticipate financial problems more often (48 percent) than men (39 percent, $\chi^2 = 3.54$, p $< .06$).

Marital status was not related to anticipated financial problems in retirement among men, indeed, 39 percent of the men expected problems regardless of marital status. Among women, however, marital status was associated with anticipated financial difficulties in retirement ($\chi^2 = 14.21$, 2 df, p $< .001$). Divorced women (60 percent) expected to be most disadvantaged followed by the widowed (48 percent), whereas never-married women (36 percent) least often anticipated difficulties and were more similar to men.

Race and Anticipated Problems in Retirement

Among women, race was associated with anticipated financial problems ($\chi^2 = 5.90$, p $< .05$) but not among men ($\chi^2 = 0$). Differences between proportions of men and women who expected problems were greater for blacks than for whites. For example, 62 percent of black women anticipated difficulties compared with 40 percent of black men, whereas comparable proportions of white men (36 percent) and white women (39 percent) were troubled about problems with money they believed they would have in retirement. Even so, in two-way analyses of variance there were no significant main effects for either anticipated problems or race on attitudes toward work or retirement for either retired men or women. Thus early anticipation of difficulties did not diminish their later endorsement of retirement as a positive decision.

Managing Anticipated Problems

Men and women who expected retirement to cause financial problems were asked how they thought they would manage. Possible responses included "receiving help from relatives," "welfare," "work a little," "don't know," and "will manage." Few men and women expected to receive help from relatives (4 and 7 percent, respectively), but even fewer anticipated they would rely on welfare, only 1 man and 3 women. Rather, most expected to work a little to make ends meet, 62 percent of the men and 60 percent of the women. About one-fifth of both sexes said they would manage without indicating how they planned to do so.

There were some differences by marital status in how persons expected to manage their financial difficulties. Among men the never married were least likely to say they would work (57 percent) compared to 69 percent of the widowed and 65 percent of the divorced. Rather, never-married men more often (30 percent) replied that they "will manage" without specifying how they planned to do so compared to about 18 percent of the formerly married men.

Widows (10 percent) expected some assistance from relatives whereas divorced women expected no help from kin. Working a little was also the most frequently expected method of managing by women although divorced women were much more likely to see work as an option, 75 percent compared to 56 percent of the widowed and never-married women. In contrast, widows and the never married were more likely to say they would manage without specifying how, 25 percent of each compared to 8 percent of the divorced. The never married more often (16 percent) than the divorced (12 percent) and widowed (9 percent) said they did not know what they would do.

Of all the sex and marital status groups, divorced women most frequently expected to manage their anticipated financial difficulties by working. This expectation was realized in that by the close of the decade more of the divorced women were employed than any other group (18 percent) even though at the beginning of the decade never-married women were more often in the labor force.

The Long Reach of Anticipated Financial Difficulties

Was the expectation of problems at the beginning of the decade reflected in financial difficulties ten years later? To answer this question, separate two-way analyses of variance were completed for retired men and women. These analyses considered the independent and potential joint effects of marital status and the earlier expectation of problems in retirement on satisfaction with level of living, financial hardship, happiness, and satisfaction with level of activity.

The expectation of financial difficulties in retirement came to fruition 10 years later for retired men and women compared to their counterparts who did not anticipate such problems. By the end of the decade both men and women who had expected problems ten years earlier were less satisfied with their level of living ($F = 33.01$, $p < .001$, men; 27.22, $p < .001$, women); had difficulty managing on their income ($F = 18.22$, $p < .01$; 31.75, $p < .001$); were less happy ($F = 9.14$, $p < .01$; 6.33, $p < .01$); and men were less satisfied with their level of activity ($F = 9.06$, $p < .01$). Relationships were especially strong between anticipated problems and later satisfaction with level of living and ability to get along on their income among both men and women.

There was a significant interaction effect between marital status and early identification of difficulties for happiness of women ($F = 3.44$, $p < .05$). The happiness of divorced women was most jeopardized by earlier expectations of financial difficulties in retirement. In fact, although divorced women as a group had the lowest scores on happiness ($\bar{X} = 2.09$), these who had not anticipated financial problems earlier enjoyed substantially greater happiness ($\bar{X} = 2.64$) in retirement than their peers who expected difficulties ($\bar{X} = 1.82$). The happiness of the divorced women who had more pleasant expectations for retirement exceeded that of widowed ($\bar{X} = 2.23$) or never-married women ($\bar{X} = 2.44$) who also had not anticipated problems. Such an effect was not observed in relation to the happiness of men.

Two-way analyses of variance indicated that in retirement, marital status differentiated only one of the evaluations of financial status—ability to get along on present income—for both men and women ($F = 3.27$, $p < .05$; 3.41, $p < .05$). Retired divorced men and women had substantially greater difficulties getting along on their income than the widowed and especially the never married. There were no significant interactions between anticipated difficulties in retirement and marital status for any of the assessments of finances or well-being.

Attitudes of retired men toward work and retirement at time 2 were not related to difficulties anticipated previously. Retired women with more favorable attitudes toward retirement at time 2, however, had expected fewer difficulties earlier in the decade ($F = 3.90$, $p < .05$).

SUMMARY AND DISCUSSION

The view that work may be substituted in some way for the absence of family ties with the consequence that retirement will be more difficult for the never married was not supported among these unmarried men and women. In fact, never-married women embraced retirement more than formerly married women. Only the findings for the formerly married provide some support for research indicating that women may welcome retirement less than do men (Schnore, 1985). Schnore, however, also found that even though women were more negative toward retirement than men, they wanted to retire earlier. For this sample though, remaining employed was a predictor of negative attitudes toward retirement among formerly married women as well as for never-married men and women.

Furthermore, never-married women more than formerly married women maintained their favorable attitudes toward retirement across the decade and were more positive in their later years. Contrary to some other research, these never-married women did not find retirement a less desirable time of life for them nor did they indicate a stronger endorsement of work. Never-married women will likely have had more sustained work histories than formerly married women, and their career fatigue (Rapoport & Rapoport, 1975) may parallel that of men and perhaps contribute to their approval of retirement. Never-married women also enjoyed more favorable economic circumstances at retirement than widowed and divorced women.

Formerly married women identified work as less important than did their male counterparts whereas never-married women were as committed to work at the end of the decade as men. Perhaps earlier family obligations, socialization experiences, or factors that initially selected them into marriage may have accounted for the somewhat lower work orientations of the formerly married women in comparison to men. At least for the formerly married, the findings parallel those of Schnore (1985), who found that older women valued work less than did men, but consequently there was no support for the observation (Veroff et al., 1981) that formerly married and never-married women more than men would find greater value fulfillment in work. Some of the difference may be accounted for by the wider range of ages studied by Veroff et al. or the measure used here may not have captured value fulfillment very well. Since marital status did not differentiate attitudes toward work within gender groups, differences between formerly married men and women but not between never-married men and women may seem puzzling. The never married were located at the extremes of their respective gender groups so that by time 2, never-married women had the most positive attitudes toward work of all women and never-married men had the least positive attitudes toward work among men, and the earlier sex differences in assessments at the beginning of the decade diminished over time.

There has been some debate about the relationship between attitudes toward work and retirement. Fillenbaum (1971) advanced the hypothesis that job attitudes would influence retirement attitudes only when work held a central organizing position in an individual's life. Reviewing previous literature, however, Schnore (1985) observed that attitude toward work has been inferred from attitudes toward a specific job. Using a more direct measure of work saliency, Schnore found it was negatively related to attitudes toward retirement. He concluded that when work was central in a person's life, then attitudes toward retirement were negative. Although remaining employed was a predictor of negative evaluations of retirement, perceptions of work and retirement were not related for these unmarried. Employment status was not associated with attitudes toward work. Other research using more indirect measures of commitment to work also found no relationship or weak relationships between commitment to work and attitudes toward retirement (Atchley, 1971; Glamser, 1976; Goudy et al., 1975). Persons, however, who continued to assign great importance to work were not less happy or seemingly disadvantaged by valuing work in old age. Work attitudes and happiness, for example, were uncorrelated for these unmarried men ($r = 00$) and women ($r = -.05$).

Compared with the never married, formerly married women seemed especially vulnerable to unhappiness. Practitioners with interests in preretirement planning may want to give special attention to these formerly married women. Since the proportions of the divorced are anticipated to increase in coming years, they warrant special consideration in retirement planning programs. Formerly married women were somewhat less happy with their lives at the beginning and end of the decade, and they also held more negative attitudes toward retirement than the never married. Defining retirement as a desirable experience was important to achieving happiness for all groups of women and never-married men. Clearly, earlier perceptions of retirement that developed while persons were still employed influenced their later attitudes toward not working.

Anticipation of financial problems ten years earlier by a substantial proportion of formerly married women, especially black women, suggested that intervention would have been of special benefit to them. Presumably consideration of both anticipated problems and attitudes toward retirement could be important aspects of preretirement planning programs. The well-being of many of the unmarried who anticipated problems was jeopardized and not just among women only. This seemed to be a durable strain in their lives across the decade and had long term implications for them. In determining which groups to target for intervention, however, it should be observed that anticipated problems had strong effects on perceptions of finances and well-being in retirement independent of race and marital status.

Sex Differences in Household Involvement of the Unmarried

INTRODUCTION

There is increasing interest in sex-role differentiation in both personality characteristics and in behavior in later life. A major focus of this chapter concerns sex differences in the management of household tasks by the unmarried and the sources of help they secured. The types of assistance received, the identity of the caregivers, and the potential strains for those giving and receiving help are discussed. The relationship between psychological well-being, personal characteristics, and involvement in household tasks also are described. To present the context from which these concerns emanate, I begin by reviewing some of the literature on sex role behavior and the likelihood of cross-sex activities in old age.

Literature from two fields is instructive in examining the sex-linked nature of household involvement in old age although neither type of research typically specifies activities of the unmarried. One research perspective is drawn primarily from psychology and often includes a self-assessment of respondents' sex role characteristics as masculine or feminine. This line of research frequently asks persons to rate themselves on adjectives that are stereotypically associated with masculinity, femininity, or are thought to be neutral.

The outcomes of these ratings are variously referred to as sex role self concept, sex role identity (Puglisi, 1983), sex role characteristics, and sex role orientation (Windle, 1986). This genre of research recently has included older subjects and others in various age cohorts in an effort to describe sex role characteristics over time and/or across the life span (Sinnott, 1986).

In the second research perspective, the tasks that older persons perform in the household are perhaps most often discussed in descriptions of marital roles, although many of the same activities of daily living are done irrespective of marital status. Yet, McBroom (1987) observed that since sex role orientation implies a sexual division of labor, the issues are probably more salient for married persons. Even so, tasks that may be differentiated by sex among the married may be performed by either men or women in households of the unmarried. Thus it might be expected that tasks undertaken by the unmarried would perhaps be less sex differentiated than those of the married.

Although some roles and activities are lost or diminish with age, many households tasks and chores necessary for daily living are continued throughout life. In the past several years social services and volunteer efforts that sponsor programs to perform some of these tasks have been extended into the homes of older people. In addition to types of health care, these programs include homemaker assistance, meals-on-wheels, chore and maintenance services. Whether the unmarried aged use household services provided by others may depend on the extent to which they are willing, have the skills, and are physically able to perform tasks typically done by the other sex. The extent of involvement in cross-sex activities may have implications for provision of services. This chapter examines the extent to which tasks in the home were sex-linked, and it identifies those activities with which unmarried persons were most likely to obtain assistance and who provided help most often. I begin by discussing sex role differentiation in later life and in involvement in the household. Because accomplishing personal and household tasks are necessary to maintain independent living and may entail securing various levels of assistance from others, I review conclusions about who provides care and the potential constraints faced by those who give and receive help.

SEX ROLE DIFFERENTIATION IN OLD AGE

Theory and research on sex roles indicate that individuals' behavior may vary depending on development, their experiences (including marital status or change in marital status), and social contingencies that may reward one type of behavior rather than another (Sinnott, 1986). Because it is learned, sex role behavior may change in response to shifts in beliefs about what is considered appropriate for a particular period of time in the life course or it may vary by historical period. Sex role behavior may be adopted and valued because it is functional at a specific time (Sinnott, 1986). Presumably acceptance of a wider variety of potential sex roles would permit an individual to be more responsive to multiple and perhaps contradictory demands of old age.

There are divergent views of sex role differentiation in old age. One perspective suggests that sex roles are reversed in later life. In what he described as the "normal unisex of later life," Gutmann (1975: 181) observed that a "massive turnover in sex roles takes place" in which men live out the characteristics of "femininity" previously denied them during the parenting years. A supposition was that women, when freed of their parental responsibilities, would exhibit more masculine traits whereas men, undergoing changes in the work-provider role, would be free to display feminine behavior (Gutmann, 1980; Nash & Feldman, 1981; Livson, 1983). Following this line of reasoning, we might expect that older men would become more passive, dependent, and less competitive, whereas women would become more assertive and dominant (Sinnott, 1977). In their test of this notion among women, Cooper and Gutmann (1987) observed differences in pre- and postempty-nest women with the latter being more self-confident, independent, assertive. Among couples, of course, it may be that the employment or educational status of the female partner is more salient in shaping sex role traits than parenting roles.

Another view is that sex roles may converge in later life indicating that both expectations for sex role differentiation and actual differentiation may decrease somewhat in old age (Lowenthal, Thurner, & Chiriboga, 1975; Minnigerode & Lee, 1978; Sinnott, 1986). Sinnot (1986) observed that the integration of masculinity and femininity has long been considered a basic task of later maturity.

Recent research indicates that older persons perceive they are expected to be androgynous, and they describe themselves in both masculine and feminine terms (Sinnott, 1986). Sex roles of older adults, as assessed by selection of descriptive adjectives, then tend to be androgynous rather than polarized. Sinnott (1986) found femininity scores of older persons were higher than those of other age cohorts that had been studied.

A frequently asked question is "What are the consequences of having sex role orientations that are masculine, feminine, or androgynous for psychological well-being in old age?" Sinnott (1986) expected to find androgyny, more than other sex role orientation, associated with successful aging. She found that an androgynous group of respondents had more positive mental health than polar groups, although those with masculine orientations reported better mental health than those with predominantly feminine descriptions. Androgynous women handled expressive and instrumental situations better, although both men and women with high feminine and low masculine orientations were more stressed and disadvantaged. Sinnott speculated that older adults are ready for role synthesis and use it to deal with situational complexity; she suggested that adults might set up long-term situations congruent with their roles, but that they were more likely to shift roles to match circumstances. In this view, the complex sex roles associated with androgyny are seen as adaptive for both the individual and society.

The conclusion that a decrease in sex role differentiation characteristic of old age is associated with greater behavioral flexibility, increased adaptation, and more successful aging is a prominent theme in the literature (Windle, 1986). Not all empirical tests, however, have provided support for these assumptions (Windle, 1986). Windle, for example, did not find that androgyny, compared with other sex role orientations, was linked with either greater cognitive flexibility or higher life satisfaction. Morgan, Affleck, & Riggs (1986) also failed to demonstrate the superiority of androgyny for mental health. Rather, low masculinity and high femininity in men was predictive of greater depression, whereas low masculinity was a correlate of depression among women.

Although Gutmann had personality characteristics in mind (e.g., passivity or aggressiveness), if the reversal in sex roles is as complete as he suggested we could also expect to see less differentiation in activities in the family and household. Attitudes toward sex roles may be becoming more egalitarian, but recent research, conducted mostly with young and middle-aged couples, demonstrates that household activities remain highly sex-linked with women performing most of the feminine tasks and men the masculine tasks (Nyguist, Slivken, Spence, & Helmrich, 1985; Whicker & Kronenfeld, 1986; Stafford, Backman, & DiBona, 1977). Although a gender-linked division of labor for household tasks is clearly evident among couples, less is known about the sex typing of household tasks among unmarried persons or the extent to which gender differences in household roles persist into old age.

HOUSEWORK IN OLD AGE

Much research and writing on household activities in old age has focused on the redistribution of household tasks and adjustment of couples during retirement. Findings from this research may be informative and have implications for studies of the older, unmarried aged as well. Despite a trend toward more egalitarian views of sex roles in general and toward housework specifically, changes in attitude are far from completely reflected in transitions in the division of labor in younger and older families (Keith & Wacker, 1988; Peters & Haldeman, 1987).

At retirement some men view the household as a place where they may reengage in socially acceptable tasks (Crawford, 1971). Some early data indicated that retired husbands increased their activity in the household although there were tasks that they were more likely to perform than others (Lipman, 1961). Retired men, like their younger counterparts, tended to be involved in more "masculine" activities such as yard work and home repairs, although they also participated in "feminine" tasks (e.g., washing dishes, cleaning, laundry).

A frequently stated concern, but one not often addressed with anything beyond speculation is whether sex role behavior in later life is a departure from what occurred earlier in the life cycle. One longitudinal study provided a glimpse of changes in the household participation of older men over a decade (Keith, 1985). Observations from 1,332 older men indicated that their participation in housework at two periods of time varied considerably by type of activity. Masculine tasks reflected in household repairs and lawn work were activities that most men performed at both times. With the exception of greater participation in gardening, most increased involvement when the men were older occurred in more feminine activities. Despite increases in the traditionally feminine activities, help with cooking, dishes, and laundry tended to be on an occasional basis (Keith, 1985).

Evidence of greater psychological androgyny in later life aside, household activities remain fairly sex-linked among couples. A further test of the gender-specific nature of household activities in old age is to examine the patterns of involvement among men and women who are not married. Regardless of the increasing numbers of singles at all stages of the life cycle, the household and family activities of the unmarried are often neglected.

Although few data are available on how the unmarried in any particular age group manage specific household tasks, researchers have examined the amount of free time and obligatory time of single men and women without children who were included in a national sample (Robinson et al., 1977). Obligatory activities entailed time spent in work, housework, and shopping. Unmarried men had 1½ more hours of free time per day than single women with comparable employment and family responsibilities. Women simply may have spent more time than men on similar tasks or more than likely men were able and willing to secure assistance from others. Although age was not controlled, the research suggested that unmarried men may either engage others to handle more of their obligatory household activities or give less attention to some of the tasks than do women.

Most of the unmarried aged are widowed. And for many, widowhood is a time in which new roles are acquired. For the first time in their lives, some women assume responsibility for the financial affairs of a household while men may increase their performance of more "feminine" housework. Household activities of men and women then might be most parallel at this stage of the life cycle. It may be, however, that men and women have differential access to sources of help or draw on different resources when they obtain assistance with household activities.

Evidence from British research suggests that not only did widowhood prompt some changes in domestic activities but that the transition may have been somewhat anticipatory beginning even before the death of the spouse (Bowling & Cartwright, 1982). With widowhood there were some gender role reversals, and although most persons had come from quite traditional households, they took on their new tasks, if not with some pleasure, at least with little negativism. Providing support once again for research indicating that men less readily embrace cross-sex tasks, widowers showed more dissatisfaction than widows with their new responsibilities. A greater proportion of widowers than widows had taken on new tasks after the death of their spouse. The researchers observed little sex differentiation in the activities undertaken by the widowed. Except for gardening and odd jobs around the house men received help with more tasks than did women (Bowling & Cartwright, 1982). Older men and women received more assistance than younger ones. In this chapter, I consider the extent to which the management of household tasks was sex-linked among unmarried males and females as it has been found to be among their married counterparts.

HOUSEWORK AND WELL-BEING

It has sometimes been assumed that women adjust easier in old age because they maintain continuity through housework that is less disjunctive with the activities of middle age (Johnson & Williamson, 1987). Following this reasoning, loss of a spouse through widowhood, divorce, or separation would represent a greater change for men, requiring housework skills they may not have and, hence, could be more stressful. Of course, other responsibilities, such as management of finances and property, may be equally disruptive for women.

It also has been implied that involvement of married men in "woman's work" may have negative consequences for their mental health by eroding their masculinity and self-esteem (Burke & Weir, 1976), whereas continued sex-typed behavior may facilitate adjustment of men in old age (Ballweg, 1967). More recent evidence, albeit obtained primarily from younger married men, suggests that increased participation at home may promote adjustment in the family and contribute to the well-being of men (Pleck, 1983). The benefits men obtain may depend somewhat on the type of task. Despite the suggestion of Oakley (1974) that housework is burdensome, repetitive, and unlikely to result in many, if any, benefits for either men or women, participation of older men in both masculine and feminine tasks was linked with greater life satisfaction whereas only involvement in masculine activities also prompted higher self-esteem (Keith, Powers, & Goudy, 1981). Involvement in both masculine and feminine activities facilitated adjustment to retirement for the fully retired but not for the partially retired. In general, the outcomes of cross-sex behavior for older men have been found to be either mostly positive or neutral and have failed to produce the negative consequences posited by some writers.

There is a temptation to conclude that the benefits derived by men who behaved less traditionally and participated more fully in the household to some degree supported the perspective that androgynous behavior may increase adaptability and may facilitate adjustment to later life transitions such as retirement. Yet, it must be observed that performance of masculine activities also was linked to a greater number of positive outcomes for males than was involvement in feminine tasks although participation in the latter did not have negative consequences (Keith, Powers, & Goudy, 1981).

Furthermore, how activities are regarded, that is, positive or negative perceptions of tasks, may mediate the effect of actual performance on well-being. Measures were not available to assess the direct impact of satisfaction with tasks or an evaluation of them on psychological well-being, but it was possible to consider the relationship between the amount of involvement in household tasks and general evaluations of life.

SOURCES OF ASSISTANCE AND CAREGIVING

Sources of assistance and caregiving that older persons may draw on as they attempt to meet their needs of daily living are the final concern in this section. When older unmarried persons are unable or unwilling to undertake certain tasks or activities, they often seek assistance and care from others. Needs are addressed through formal or informal ties that the older person has been able to establish.

Streib (1983) observed that because the very old do not operate as individuals who live autonomously and independently as has been assumed by traditional survey researchers, they should be considered in terms of the concept of networks or social contexts. Those who assist the aged, however, are not always clearly identified in the literature.

Research assessing the amount and/or sources of assistance with tasks of daily living in old age has not employed comparable labels, definitions, or measures. Those who provide help to the aged with tasks ranging from highly personal activities to lawn mowing have been identified as informal-formal systems (Brody, Johnsen, & Fulcomer, 1984; Circirelli, 1981), informal support networks (Morris & Sherwood, 1983–84), natural support systems (Sivley & Fiegener, 1984), social support (Bankoff, 1983), informal helpers (Stoller, 1983), intergenerational exchange when help is provided by kin (Johnson, 1983; Lee & Ellithorpe, 1982), and caregivers (Brody, 1981). Noting the lack of clarity implied in usage of the term "social support," House (1984) described it as the flow between people of emotional concern, instrument aid, information, or appraisal.

Research on older persons and their families documents the persistence of intergenerational ties, sustained and extensive contact between parents and adult children, the importance of the family in caring for the elderly who need help (Stoller, 1983), and the resistance of families to placing their older members in institutions (Brody, 1981; Shanas, 1979). Estimates of the amount of care provided by helpers vary, although it is suggested that from one-fourth to one-third of the aged living in the community require assistance with home care (Brody, 1981). The preference is for care in the community; kin (usually children), friends, and neighbors are viewed as the most appropriate caregivers in the majority of situations (Cantor, 1980).

Even among the most frail, unless health is almost completely eroded, assistance is primarily provided outside a formal organization (Cantor, 1980). Indeed, a minority of the aged being cared for in the community are more disabled than those in institutions. Thus the availability of caregivers may be as important as the person's level of functioning in determining institutionalization. Persons with less access to caregivers, especially the unmarried, are more likely to be institutionalized even though they may have fewer medical problems and lower levels of disability than persons with adequate helpers (Morris & Sherwood, 1984).

Within the family, a spouse (if available) assumes the major caregiving tasks, often precluding institutionalization for the disabled partner (Palmore, 1976). Of course, the very old are more likely to be unmarried or the spouse is also more apt to be frail. Among the widowed and the divorced with children, a child (usually a daughter) most often provides care. Most comprehensive and long-term care is provided by children, but siblings, kin, friends, neighbors, and formal organizations also assist (Cantor, 1980). Family members may deliver as much as 80 percent of the home health care provided to older persons (Morris & Sherwood, 1983-84).

Comprehensive care, however, is provided in descending order of kinship; the spouse provides the most complete care, efforts of children are less extensive, and more distant kin and nonkin give the least amount of assistance (Johnson, 1983). In the absence of a spouse or child, assistance provided by other relatives tends to be more perfunctory (Johnson & Catalano, 1981). Johnson (1983) found little sharing of functions between kin. The family and formal organizations share care more often for the unmarried, especially those without children.

TWO CONTRASTING VIEWS OF THE RESOURCES OF CAREGIVERS AND HELPERS

There are two contrasting views of those who provide care to the aged living in the community. One theme stresses the responsiveness of family members, friends, and neighbors to the needs of older persons (Morris & Sherwood, 1983-84; Johnson, 1983; Wenger, 1981). This view calls attention to the proximity of and frequent contact with children, endorsement of filial obligation by offspring (Seelbach, 1978), and the willingness of friends and neighbors to provide assistance in crisis situations as well as more sustained caregiving activities (Morris & Sherwood, 1983–84; Wenger, 1981). The informal support system is described as resilient, is projected to remain elastic, and "will not be affected adversely by the assumption of unanticipated roles" (Morris & Sherwood, 1983–84). Informal caregivers are viewed as having a great deal of response capability to manage decreases in the functional capacities of the vulnerable elderly (Morris & Sherwood, 1983–84). In this perspective, caregivers and helpers are viewed as readily available and responsive to the unexpected needs of the aged with minimal strain.

There are, however, demographic and social changes that may limit the capacity of informal caregivers in the future. "At the same time as the proportion of the elderly population requiring care is expanding, other demographic and social changes, including the decline in the birth rate, delay in the age of parenthood, increase in divorce and in single-parent families and most importantly, the growth in the labor market activity of women, have reduced the pool of potential caregivers" (Finch & Groves, 1983).

With these demographic and social changes in mind, a second perspective acknowledges the vulnerability, competing commitment, strain, and limitations of informal caregivers (Johnson, 1983; Brody, 1981; Finch & Groves, 1983). This perspective suggests that tasks of caregivers are added to the multiple role demands that middle-aged women, who tend to be the primary caregivers, already have. Women confront competing demands as employee, wife, mother, and daughter to frail parents. That caregiving may be added to other tasks is evidenced by the finding that whereas the employment status of men diminished the amount of care they gave, caregiving by women was not associated with the amount of time they spent in the labor force (Stoller, 1983).

Strain experienced by caregivers may affect relationships with their spouses and other family members, plans for their own retirement, be accompanied by the emotional burden of anticipating their parent's further decline, and perhaps their own and/or their spouse's failing health. There is some evidence that providing long-term care may exacerbate a number of health problems of the caregiver (Crossman, London, & Barry, 1981). In this perspective, the well-being of both caregivers and the aged is perceived as potentially under threat. When they need assistance, the unmarried cannot rely on a spouse and for 20 percent more children are not available. This suggests that friends and formal organizations may be especially critical.

It is likely that attributes such as health, age, socioeconomic status, and the presence of family and friends will influence the unmarried in seeking help from others. Moreover, these characteristics may differentially affect the activities of men and women. In this chapter, health, age, income, education, and the number and proximity of family and friends as potential sources of help are investigated in relation to the household activities and needs of unmarried men and women.

This chapter then addresses four questions: To what extent are unmarried men and women involved in different household tasks in old age? How do they manage household activities they do not perform themselves? Does household involvement contribute to well-being or is it especially disadvantageous for men? Are the personal characteristics associated with household involvement comparable for men and women?

PROCEDURES

Sample

Because household activities and assistance attained from others are important to the maintenance of independent living and because information on involvement in the home was not collected in the Retirement History Study, data from another longitudinal study with a sample of unmarried aged were analyzed for this chapter. Data were obtained from structured interviews conducted with 55 men and 286 women during the second phase of a longitudinal study of the aged in small towns. Respondents resided in towns of 250 to 5,000 in a midwestern state. In the initial study, 1,700 respondents were randomly selected from a sample of towns drawn to be representative of small towns in the state.

To determine the household roles that men and women undertook in the absence of a spouse, persons who were widowed, divorced, or separated were studied. Because most of the unmarried persons in the total sample had been married previously and because sex roles developed in a marriage may continue to influence how household tasks are managed when a person becomes single again, the small number of never-married individuals (n = 22) were excluded. The data analyzed then are based on a previously married subsample of the total sample of 568 individuals interviewed in the second wave of a longitudinal study. For brevity, respondents will be referred to as unmarried.

Although the sample was not assumed to be representative of unmarried men and women age 65 or over, the sex distribution of the subsample was identical to that of the population in this age group in the United States in which 16 percent of all males 65 years or over were widowed or divorced compared with 56 percent of the women at the time the data were obtained. Respondents ranged in age from 72 to 97 with a median age of 80.

Education, Income, and Health

Education was coded in number of years, and over half of the sample had eight or less years of education. Income was coded in six categories ranging from less than $1,000 per year to $15,000 or more per year. About 70 percent had incomes of less than $3,000. Health was measured by the question: "How is your health generally?" with 40 percent reporting "good" (3), 38 percent "fair" (2) and 22 percent "poor" (1).

Household Activities

To measure involvement in household activities, respondents indicated whether they did the following household tasks for themselves, or whether someone else did them: laundry, writing letters or bills, running errands outside the house, shopping, yard work and repairs, meals, and other housework. A household tasks score was obtained by summing the number of activities that an individual performed. The theoretical range of scores was from zero to seven with a high score indicating greater household involvement.

Life Satisfaction

Life satisfaction was assessed by ten items (see Wood et al., 1969 for these items). Response categories were agree, disagree, and do not know. Scores were obtained by summing across the ten items with higher scores indicating greater life satisfaction. The coefficient of reliability was .67 (Alpha).

Family and Friends

Respondents indicated the number of living children, grandchildren, siblings, total number of friends, and number of close friends they had. They were coded so that a larger number indicated a greater number of relatives and friends. Respondents also identified the physical proximity of each of the following: their closest child, closest relative other than a child, and that of their closest friend. These were coded with 1 indicating the person lived on the same street or in the neighborhood and ranged to 7 which represented a distance of more than 100 miles. These factors were used to assess availability of potential sources of help.

RESULTS

There was little evidence to support a norm of unisex household involvement among the widowed in old age (Table 7.1). In fact there was considerable divergence in the tasks performed by men and women. In five of the seven tasks, men and women differed in their involvement with women performing four of the seven more frequently. Amount of participation varied by task as well as by sex. For example, over 80 percent of the women did their own cooking

Table 7.1

Number and Percentage of Men and Women Involved in Household Activities

Task	Men (n=55)		Women (n=286)		χ^2	p
	N	%	N	%		
Laundry	24	44	182	64	6.90	.01
Correspondence (Letters & Bills)	34	62	240	84	12.90	.001
Errands (outside the house)	32	58	157	55	.09	ns
Shopping	29	53	149	52	.00	ns
Yard Work & Home Repairs	28	51	53	19	24.94	.001
Cooking	36	66	243	85	10.53	.001
Housework	30	54	207	72	6.10	.01

and handled their correspondence compared with a little over 60 percent of the men. In comparison with cooking and correspondence, fewer women, however, did their own laundry (64 percent) and housework (72 percent). Although men were substantially less involved in these tasks, their patterns of participation were the same with fewer doing laundry (44 percent) and other housework (54 percent). Men clearly made more alternative arrangements for handling some of the "feminine" activities than did women.

Men and women did not differ in the degree to which they managed their own errands and shopping. Household repairs and yard work were the most sex-linked activities with only 19 percent of the women ever performing these tasks whereas about 50 percent of the men were involved.

Since tasks remain sex-linked among the unmarried aged, did men and women seek different sources of help when they did not assume responsibility for the activities themselves? Although the numbers tended to be small in some of the categories of sources of help, they were suggestive of how the old who were unmarried managed their lives. Sources of help primarily included children, friends, and hired persons with less assistance from grandchildren, siblings, and more distant relatives. Children provided the most help to both sexes although on most tasks men tended to rely somewhat more on children than did women. Women, however, received help with yard work from children far more frequently (21 percent) than did men (2 percent). In all activities except cooking and housekeeping, women tended to depend more on hired services. On the other hand, men received more help from their friends. Although grandchildren rarely assisted with any household activities, they helped men with repairs and yard work (11 percent) more than they helped women (3 percent). Siblings, however, were seldom sources of help for either sex on the activities considered.

This raised a question about the availability of each of the potential sources of help. For the most part, men and women differed little in their access to family members. For example, the proportions of men and women without living children or with no children in the same town were comparable. Men, however, were more likely (54 percent) to have close relatives other than children living in the same town than were women (40 percent). Men were less likely to have close friends and/or had fewer friends than did women. Yet over two-thirds of the men and women who identified close friends had a friend who lived in close proximity (next door, on the same street, or in the neighborhood).

Although men and women generally had comparable access to potential sources of help, correlations between avilability and proximity of individual potential support systems and the cumulative housework scores indicated that the sources were differentially related to the household activities of unmarried men and women. For example, having children (r = −.22), grandchildren (r = −.22), and their location (r = .31) in the same town all influenced the degree of male household involvement. As might be expected, men with fewer children or whose children or other relatives were located farther away were responsible for more of their own household tasks. The total number of friends (r = .05), the number of close friends (r = .05), and proximity of the closest friend (r = −.05), however, made no difference in the household involvement of men.

Women with more children (r = −.12) and whose children lived closer (r = .14) tended to assume less responsibility for their household tasks. But women with more brothers and sisters (r = .14), a greater total number of friends (r = .16) and more close friends (r = .14) tended to do more of their own household tasks. Number of grandchildren (r = .01) and proximity of the closest friend (r = −.01) did not affect women's participation in the household.

The correlations between potential sources of help and household involvement for women generally were lower than those for men. On six of the eight measures, there was a .10 or greater difference in the correlations between potential sources of help and the assistance obtained by men and those of women. Five of the measures of sources of help involved family members or their proximity to the older person. On all but one of these (number of siblings), relationships between types of help and household involvement were stronger for men than for women. For the most part, however, the relationships were only suggestive of potential differences in the ways unmarried men and women managed to accomplish activities of daily living.

These men tended to draw on family for help to a greater extent than did women. On two of the three measures pertaining to friends (i.e., number and proximity) relationships between potential source of help and involvement were stronger for women than for men. Rather than friends being sought as sources of help and diminishing the amount of work done by women, those with more friends were more involved in their own household. Probably, women who were able to maintain friendship ties were also physically more able to run their household.

A remaining question concerns the consequences of household involvement for psychological well-being in old age. Was the well-being of men and women differentially influenced by participation in housework? Were unmarried men disadvantaged when they assumed responsibility for their household activities?

Men who were responsible for more of their own housework and performed more feminine tasks were not disadvantaged and were as well-adjusted as those who were less involved in the household. In fact, even though relationships between the cumulative household involvement scores and evaluations of life were not strong, they were positive for both men ($r = .17$) and women ($r = .16$).

In summary, it is clear that men and women were involved in somewhat different tasks in old age, that beyond receiving help from children they obtained assistance from somewhat different sources, and both sexes derived some benefit from involvement in housework. A further question was the extent to which different personal characteristics seemed to foster involvement in the household among men and women.

Health did not differ significantly for men and women. Women were somewhat older than men, but age and health were not related. Health, age, education, and income were examined in relation to household involvement for men and women.

In a multiple regression analysis, health accounted for the most variance in the household involvement of men ($r = .42$; $b = .47$). Men who were in better health were more involved in the household. Although age and education were included in the regression equation, they were weakly correlated with household participation ($r = -.12$; 17, respectively). The three variables explained 22 percent of the variance in involvement. The correlation between income and household involvement was .16 for men, but when other variables were considered, finances did not directly influence participation.

Age and health were of about equal importance in accounting for the household involvement of women. Women who were younger ($r = .42$; $b = .38$) and in better health ($r = .38$; $b = .34$) were more involved. These variables explained 29 percent of the variance. Neither education ($r = .08$) nor income ($r = .05$) contributed significantly to the involvement of women.

Even though men and women were engaged in somewhat different activities in old age, health was a significant factor in determining the household participation of both. Furthermore, income was not salient in the household involvement of either men or women. The unimportance of income probably reflected the tendency to obtain volunteer help from family members or unpaid assistance from others.

SUMMARY AND DISCUSSION

A "normal unisex pattern" posited to occur in late life indicates that we might find men and women behaving very much the same in old age. Certainly sex roles had not merged to the point that these older men and women performed household activities to the same extent. Even the absence of a spouse did not eliminate the sex-linked characteristics of housework in old age although life changes including the acquisition of new roles in widowhood are frequently assumed to include more cross-sex tasks.

The consequences of cross-sex behavior in old age are unclear, but androgyny is often thought to be linked with greater adaptive capacities or at least not negative (Sinnott, 1986). Some research, however, indicates that sex-linked reversals in personal characteristics may have different consequences for males and females (Frank, Towell, & Huyck, 1985). For example, low masculinity was associated with depression in females (Morgan, Affleck, & Riggs, 1986) whereas a more feminine orientation was linked to poorer ratings of mental health among both men and women (Frank, Towell, & Huyck, 1985). Other research indicated that women who more closely resembled older males were more successful in old age, but males who "maintained a dominant aggressive stance" were more successful than their peers who manifested greater cross-sex behavioral characteristics (Lieberman, 1978).

Among these very old men, however, performance of cross-sex tasks did not result in negative evaluations of life. In fact, those men who performed a variety of household tasks in the absence of a spouse derived some benefit from it. Although data were not available to determine whether participation of men was higher than when their spouses were alive, in all likelihood they had become more involved and acquired some new roles in widowhood. Certainly the profile of the older widower alone and bereft of any social ties that could provide assistance in the household was not evident; in fact, corroborating other research (Beattie, 1976), men were more likely to receive support services from friends and kin than were women. Single men may define themselves or be seen by others as being less adept at household activities than women are and consequently have more friends and family who are eager to help a male in need of domestic assistance.

It may be that involvement in housework in old age represents engagement and hence, any negative effects of participation in "feminine" activities or "woman's work" by men might be offset by the sheer benefits of involvement. For some men who are alone, "woman's work" may be about the only work remaining to be done. Indeed, the very kinds of tasks sometimes so maligned by younger persons as overload, routine, and demoralizing may represent independence for the very old of either sex. The assumption that women may be better able to adjust to retirement and old age because they can maintain continuity in their lives through involvement in household activities (Johnson & Williamson, 1987) received little support. In fact, the data indicated that the well-being of these women was not contingent on involvement in the household to any greater degree than that of men. In general, although women were more involved than men, the benefits, if any, from their participation in household activities did not result in more positive evaluations of life.

Health was the only personal factor that was a determinant of involvement of both men and women. Age had an independent influence on the participation of women but not of men. Although the data indicated that the gender-linked nature of household activities persisted into very late life, future research may reveal further differences as well. Males and females also may vary in their competency in performing household tasks and in the enjoyment they obtain from the roles.

This research suggested that unmarried men needed considerably more assistance with activities performed inside the home than did women. These are usually regarded as feminine tasks that require some time every day and are generally more time consuming on a regular basis (Beckman & Houser, 1979). Needs of unmarried men for assistance with household activities have implications for both formal and informal sources of help. Needs that have to be met on a daily basis are, for the most part, more demanding than those that require only occasional attention. The predominant needs of men, more than those of women, will likely intrude more into the lives of their families if they provide help or men may use more agency resources for household assistance if such services are available.

When help was obtained, both men and women used mostly informal sources with reliance primarily on children and to a lesser degree friends (Wenger, 1981). Further examination of the management of household roles by the aged should explore in some detail how patterns of intergenerational helping and assistance influence parent-child relationships in adulthood and whether they differ for unmarried men and women compared to their counterparts in couples.

Lee (1985) observed that older persons believed that professional (formal) services could replace those contributed by family members, and that they would rather pay for this assistance than request help from kin. Indeed, older persons expected and desired less help from kin than younger individuals were prepared to give. Endorsing norms of greater independence seemed to have positive outcomes. Other research has indicated that receiving assistance from relatives may have detrimental consequences for mental health. For example, regardless of marital status, persons who expected assistance from a child expressed less happiness (Lee, 1985). Lee suggested that assistance from formal sources be increased rather than encouraging additional support from those with whom informal ties are maintained.

Future research also may include investigation of the way in which patterns of helping established by friends affect interaction as well as the meaning of and changes in the informal relationship between those who help and those who receive assistance. Interaction with friends usually contributes more to the psychological well-being of the aged than contact with family (Lee, 1985). But we need to know how sustained helping relationships and possibly dependency affect the outcomes of these social ties.

Use of Time: Continuity and Change **8**

Robinson (1977) observed that what people do with their time is of concern to every society and especially in industrialized countries in which the regulation and use of time is central to assessments of societal functioning. At the individual level, how time is spent also has a bearing on the quality of life. Increased longevity and earlier retirement are creating unprecedented leisure options for older persons. For retirees, the additional time they have probably represents one of the immediate major changes in their lives.

For most older persons, retirement brings increased free time and for many it is a contrast with the busyness of fulltime work outside the home. It has sometimes been assumed, although not always strongly supported, that the consequences of withdrawing from or reducing activities will be negative. There has been concern about the consequences of doing very little, but significantly less attention has been given to exactly how older persons spend their time. Even though only a small percentage of older persons observe that they have too much "time on their hands," some express solicitude that the retired may "waste" their time or that they will decline physically or mentally because they have nothing to do (Foner & Schwab, 1981).

Whereas the consequences of continuity, reduction, replacement, or increases in activities in later life have been the source of considerable speculation and hypothesis testing over the last several years in social gerontology, beyond the major life roles (e.g., marital status, employment) that determine how people allocate some of their hours, less is known about how persons spend their time when work and a spouse may no longer figure in their lives or perhaps have never been a factor. What is known is that most persons do not find new activities when they retire (Foner, 1986). Some research demonstrated that leisure behavior characterizing persons during their working lives continued almost unchanged (Kremer & Harpaz, 1982). Furthermore, advantaged circumstances did not have much effect on changes in the use of leisure. Having good health, financial security, and abundant free time did not seem to foster new ways of using time or result in the initiation of further creative activities.

In general, leisure in later life tends to reflect continuity with earlier adult periods (Kelly, Steinkamp, & Kelly, 1986). Adults have a core of leisure activities that persists throughout the life course (Kelly et al., 1986). There is evidence that retirees also maintain stable views of themselves as leisure participants (Bosse & Ekerdt, 1981). A comparison of recent retirees and persons who remained in the labor force revealed that the former did not perceive they had increased amounts of leisure involvement. Furthermore, the retired did not view themselves as more involved in leisure activities than age peers who were still employed. Thus literature suggests there is continuity in type and amount of leisure pursuits in pre- and post-retirement as well as little perceived change in these activities with retirement. To the extent that early patterns of activities predict later participation, leisure involvement then should be conceptualized as a lifelong process that will be maintained consistently throughout the life cycle unless poor health or other circumstances become barriers to participation (Bosse & Ekerdt, 1981). In studies of leisure across the life span it has been observed that if there are changes with age, leisure participation is increasingly passive and homebound (Roadburg, 1981).

Most activities are undertaken in or near the residence and are an integral aspect of ongoing daily life. Some of these family, social, home-based and out-of-home leisure pursuits and changes in them over a period of years are the focus of this chapter. In this chapter, I consider informal social ties with kin and friends, participation in formal organizations, and leisure activities that may or may not involve interaction with others. The activities studied here are pursued in and out of the home; they also differ in cost and expenditure of energy. First, I examine the prevalence of social ties and activities, changes in them over a decade, and how they varied by gender and marital status. Isolation from others and correlates of affiliation with children, siblings and friends are considered. Factors associated with participation in formal organizations are discussed in Chapter 9.

KIN AND FRIENDS OF THE UNMARRIED

Stein (1976) observed that the greatest need expressed by singles is for networks of social relationships that can facilitate sharing, intimacy, and continuity, needs presumably met by the marital partnership. Singles would have to meet these outside of marriage. Support from friendships may be salient "particularly for those who lack institutional roles because they are retired, widowed, or single" (Ward, 1984).

Although some research has compared ties of the married and unmarried, little is available that systematically compares the social relationships of specific groups of the unmarried aged. Representative research (Ward, 1979; Babchuck, 1978–79) has considered the number and/or frequency of contact with kin and friends by marital status. It would be expected that the unmarried would vary in their access to family members especially since the majority of the never married would not have children, and divorce may alter patterns of interaction with kin (Hennon, 1983). Since the availability of family members is presumed to provide opportunities for interaction with others, clearly some groups are at greater risk of isolation than others. Those who are aged, unmarried, and childless may be especially vulnerable to isolation.

Persons may compensate for the absence of a spouse and children by affiliating with relatives. For example, in one study it was found that over half (55 percent) of the childless aged had seen a sibling or other relative within the previous week (Shanas, 1979), and 43 percent of never-married older persons had face-to-face contact with a sibling within the previous 24 hours compared with only 6 percent of the formerly married (Willmott & Young, 1960). In contrast, Babchuck (1978–79) found that the formerly married, along with the married, had a greater number of primary kin and confidants than the never married. Ward (1979) also observed that never-married persons were less likely to see relatives on a weekly or daily basis than are the formerly married.

Among the unmarried, the quality of family ties varies by sex and marital status; divorced men were less satisfied than never-married or widowed men, but differences were small among unmarried women. Ward concluded that the dissolution of marriage affects the quality of family life of men more than that of women (Ward, 1979).

It is possible that the never married might compensate for their lower family contact by maintaining a greater number of ties with friends. However, Babchuck observed that although never-married persons had fewer primary and confidant kin, they had no more primary or confidant friends than those who had been married. But Ward, using a national sample, and Atchley, Pignatiello, and Shaw (1979) reported greater contact with friends by the never married than by the married.

Several studies indicate that widows at least seemed to maintain larger networks than married women (Anderson, 1984; Kohen, 1983). In a study of women only, the married, regardless of occupation, had less yearly interaction with friends than widowed women (Atchley, Pignatiello, & Shaw, 1979). Ward also observed less daily or weekly contact with neighbors and other friends by married men and women than by any category of the unmarried. Supporting the view that the marital dyad may be the primary focus for the married whereas the absence of a spouse may enhance ties with others, Kohen (1983) concluded that widowed women maintained more contact with kin, friends, and neighbors than did the married.

Gender, however, was again a factor in shaping social relationships since the ties of both widowed and married women exceeded those of married or widowed men (Kohen, 1983; Longino & Lipman, 1981). Widowers were especially bereft of primary contacts (Longino & Lipman, 1981) and saw less of their friends than widows (Arens, 1982–83). Whereas widowhood may stimulate women to expand their ties and form new relationships, widowers coped by retaining the familiar social networks they relied on when their spouses were alive (Hyman, 1983). One source of contact with others especially for widowers was with service providers (Longino & Lipman, 1981). Among men and women in planned retirement communities, Longino and Lipman (1981) concluded that the married had more primary relations that provided support, and those without spouses had more secondary relations.

It is somewhat unclear how marital status will differentiate the social activities of the unmarried. Ward (1979) reported that the unmarried—the widowed, divorced/separated, or never married— differed little in the frequency with which they saw neighbors or other friends on a weekly or daily basis. Hyman (1983), however, observed variation in the social lives of widowed and divorced women. Widows were more likely to spend a social evening with relatives (45 percent) once a week or more often than were divorced women (33 percent), although the latter spent a little more time with friends. More divorced women (41 percent) had no involvement in voluntary associations or never attended church services (20 percent) than widows (31 percent; 10 percent, respectively). Hyman (1983) noted that more informal social relationships outside the family were maintained by older divorced and separated men than by the widowed. More divorced men, for example, spent a social evening with neighbors at least once a week (42 percent) than did widowers (30 percent). Divorced men also frequented bars/taverns much more often (33 percent weekly or more often) than widowed men (9 percent), but they were less active in formal organizations. Forty-eight percent maintained no memberships in voluntary associations compared to 32 percent of the widowers who had no affiliation with formal organizations. The greater isolation of the divorced men from formal community organizations also was reflected in their nonattendance at religious services; 36 percent never attended compared to 16 percent of the widowers. In the main, Hyman commented on the marked negative effect of divorce or separation on the social lives of unmarried men.

Thus limited data suggest that among older people the married may have more contact with kin although the unmarried maintain more ties with friends. Among the unmarried the widowed seem to keep in touch with kin more than the divorced. The never married appear to have less contact with kin than the formerly married, but it is less clear how relationships with friends differ among the formerly married and never married. For the formerly married who have experienced loss of a spouse, it is likely that previous involvement with family, friends, and in organizations would remain the best predictor of relationships after the change in status.

PERSONAL CHARACTERISTICS AND SOCIAL TIES

Personal characteristics such as income, education, health, and employment status potentially may influence social ties in old age. With the exception of education, these attributes may undergo considerable change in later life.

In general, persons of low socioeconomic status, low income, and less education have smaller social networks, often consisting primarily of family members (Antonucci, 1985). Babchuck (1978–79), how-ever, concluded that persons with more schooling and in higher occu-pations had richer networks of *both* friends and kin and were less isolated from relatives than is sometimes implied in the literature. Furthermore, working-class persons did not limit themselves to fam-ily members as is sometimes suggested.

The literature includes competing hypotheses about the relation-ship between affiliation and retirement. One view indicates the retired will compensate for their loss of ties at work by stepping up their levels of activity outside the workplace. However, a rival view might posit that retirement will diminish a major source of friend-ships, perhaps especially for the unmarried who may rely more on the workplace to provide opportunities for socializing.

The bulk of evidence indicates that persons at least maintain previous levels of social activity following retirement (Walker et al., 1980–81) although Atchley (1976) found that men assumed they would increase interaction in retirement. In general, however, there seems to be continuity in social networks in pre- and postretirement (Antonucci, 1985). Finally, health has a significant influence on engaging in activities with family and friends by older persons (Roberto & Scott, 1986).

SOCIAL RELATIONS AND WELL-BEING

To place the examination of relationships with family and friends in context, it is important to determine the consequences of informal social ties in old age. Do those with social ties fare better than their isolated peers? In general, informal social relationships are believed to promote psychological well-being in later life (see Chown, 1981, for a review). Although some research fails to find a relationship be-tween number of friends, amount of contact with friends, and well-being (e.g., morale, happiness, or satisfaction), several studies of older persons have found that friends seem to foster positive outlooks on life (Chown, 1981; Edwards & Klemmack, 1973; Lee, 1985; Veen-hoven, 1984). Interaction with family members, however, may con-tribute less to psychological well-being than do friends (Chown, 1981; Lee, 1985). In the next chapter, the contribution of activities to the happiness of the unmarried in rural and urban places is studied.

CONTACT WITH CHILDREN

The importance of children in the social lives of most older persons is undisputed. To dispel myths of an elderly population abandoned by their children, the frequent contact between them is often noted (Lee, 1985). For many persons, ties with immediate family members are somewhat more prevalent than those with friends and neighbors. The majority of older persons have frequent contact with a child; for example 75 percent see one child at least weekly (Ward, 1984). Indeed, the availability of children for affiliation and assistance is a major factor differentiating the social lives of many of the formerly married from most of the never married. Children especially may provide support to the aged without spouses who tend to rely more on them than do married couples.

CHILDLESSNESS AND ISOLATION FROM CHILDREN BY THE FORMERLY MARRIED

Having no children or not associating with those who are available may have some comparable outcomes in old age, that is, an absent source of potential support for tasks of daily living or help in illness and a greater probability of social isolation (Bachrach, 1980). In Chapter 10 on the vulnerable elderly, unmarried parents and the childless are compared in more detail.

Nationally about 20 percent of the older population have no living children. In the general population, childless people include married couples who had no children (intentionally or involuntarily), widowed and divorced with no children, and the never married without children. In old age, a minority of the unmarried childless will have lost children through death, but the majority would never have had them.

Corresponding to national data by time 2, a little over one-fifth of the divorced men (22 percent) and women (21 percent) and almost that many widowed women (18 percent) had no living children (Table 8.1). Somewhat fewer widowed men had no children, 14 percent. Most had been childless over the decade.

These widowed men and women had a greater number of living children than the divorced. Widowed men had the most, averaging 2.7 whereas widowed women had slightly fewer, 2.4. Divorced men and women had an average of two living children, although the averages obscure the substantial minority with no children.

Table 8.1
Availability and Absence of Contact with Children/Siblings
by Time, Sex, and Marital Status

	Men		Women	
	Time 1	Time 2	Time 1	Time 2
% No Children				
Widowed	13	14	17	18
Divorced	20	22	20	21
% No Contact with Children				
Widowed	21	17	20	10
Divorced	23	23	16	11
% No Siblings				
Widowed	8	10	11	17
Divorced	5	12	12	20
Never Married	7	13	11	16
% No Contact with Siblings				
Widowed	10	10	12	12
Divorced	17	15	12	18
Never Married	8	15	11	17

Having children, however, did not ensure that relationships would be such that they and their parents would see one another. From 10 to over 20 percent of the formerly married did not have any contact with children in person or by phone, and there was variation in contact by gender. By time 2, relationships of widowed and divorced men with their children were quite different from those of formerly married women; almost twice as many men as women were estranged from children and never contacted them (Table 8.1). For example, 23 percent of the divorced men never saw or spoke with their children by phone compared to 11 percent of the divorced women. Contact with children by divorced men was considerably lower than that reported by Shanas (1979) who found that 13 percent of the men and 9 percent of women had not seen a child for longer than one month although she did not consider differences by marital status.

Combining the percentage of persons without children with those who had no contact may give some notion of the proportion of the unmarried elderly who might not be able to count on children for any kind of sustained support. Divorced men were least likely to be able to look to children for assistance. Forty-five percent of the divorced men either had no children or no contact with them compared to about 30 percent of the other formerly married men and women. Most of the difference in the isolation from children experienced by divorced men and the other formerly married was attributable to the failure of divorced men to maintain contact with living children. To the degree that children may be a resource in later life, a substantial minority of these unmarried would have to rely on resources other than children, but divorced men especially would need to seek out other sources of help and affiliation.

MARITAL STATUS, GENDER, AND AMOUNT OF CONTACT WITH CHILDREN

Among the majority who did see children, marital status and gender differentiated the extent of their ties. Persons indicated the frequency with which they had contact with children ranging from "Daily, Weekly, Monthly, Less than monthly, or Never."

Widowed men tended to see or phone children more often than divorced men both earlier and later in their lives ($t = 1.74$, $p < .10$; 2.32, $p < .05$). Despite their greater number of children, widowed women did not differ from divorced women in the frequency with which they had contact with children at either the beginning or the end of the decade ($t = .58$; 1.39).

Over the decade, gender was linked to affiliation with children with women having the most contact. Both when they were younger and older, divorced women saw children more than divorced men ($t = 3.13$, $p < .01$; $t = 4.55$, $p < .001$), whereas the greatest differences between widowed men and women occurred later in their lives ($t = 1.46$, ns; $t = 2.57$, $p < .01$, time 1 and time 2, respectively). Thus formerly married men were less likely than women to see children frequently, and among those with at least some contact with children divorced men were most isolated from theirs.

CHANGE IN CONTACT WITH CHILDREN

Literature seeking to document that elders may be abandoned by their children when they are old again received little support, although

Table 8.2
Change in Amount of Contact with Children, Siblings, and Friends
from Time 1 to Time 2 by Sex and Marital Status

		Percent of Those Who Changed	
	% Change	% Increase	% Decrease
Men/Children			
Widowed	38	62	38
Divorced	28	50	50
Women/Children			
Widowed	28	62	38
Divorced	29	57	43
Men/Siblings			
Widowed	30	26	74
Divorced	24	22	78
Never Married	25	37	63
Women/Siblings			
Widowed	26	43	57
Divorced	28	26	74
Never Married	33	38	62
Men/Friends			
Widowed	42	20	80
Divorced	43	18	82
Never Married	45	38	62
Women/Friends			
Widowed	33	22	78
Divorced	36	23	77
Never Married	27	29	71

time spent with children changed over the decade for more than one quarter of these formerly married men and women (Table 8.2). Indeed, isolation from children generally decreased. Widowed men more often (38 percent) experienced change in the amount of time spent with their children compared to 28 percent of the divorced men. Furthermore, of the widowed men who changed their affiliation over the decade, 62 percent increased their ties with children whereas divorced men were as likely to become isolated from their children as to increase the amount of time spent with them (50 percent).

More than one quarter of widowed and divorced women (28, 29 percent) changed their interaction with children over the decade. The majority of those who changed increased their ties with children (62 percent, widowed; 57 percent, divorced).

An important thing to keep in mind is that for most of the unmarried (70 percent), ties with children were stable over time. For the majority of those who changed, the transition resulted in closer contact with children.

CORRELATES OF CHANGE IN CONTACT WITH CHILDREN

What factors seemed to make a difference in whether unmarried parents increased, decreased, or maintained the same amount of contact with their children? To what extent did personal characteristics foster changes in affiliation with children? Health, education, income, and employment status were examined in relation to whether ties with children had increased, decreased or remained the same. Personal characteristics at both the beginning and end of the decade were largely unrelated to the pattern of changes among women although divorced and widowed women who were in poorer health at time 1 ($r = -.16$) and time 2 ($r = -.12$), respectively, increased their contact with children somewhat. Both initially and later in their lives widowers in better health, however, saw more of their children ($r = .16$, time 1; .18, time 2). Speculation that a parent's poor health may prompt increased contact with children in old age received little sustained support over time and across marital statuses.

Higher income at both the beginning and end of the decade was associated with increased interaction with children by widowed men ($r = .18$; .18) and by divorced men at time 2 ($r = .16$). In summary, widowers' patterns of interaction with children were influenced most consistently by health and income. Access to children by women was less affected by their economic status. Education and employment status did not either foster or curtail change in interaction with children. Indeed, of the 32 correlations (i.e., four variables [health, income, education, employment] X four gender-marital status groups X two interviews) only the seven modest relationships mentioned above were larger than $r = .10$. For the most part, among these formerly married men and women change in interaction with their children was independent of health, employment, and dimensions of socioeconomic status.

THE LONG REACH OF SIBLING TIES

A number of conditions differentiate sibling relationships from those established with others (Cicirelli, 1982). Relationships between siblings potentially may be the longest family tie one can experience beginning at birth and well before marriage or parenthood. Siblings usually share childhood and an environment emphasizing common values. In this setting they may have a highly egalitarian relationship (compared to the parent-child bond). Experiences with siblings provide an anchor in a common history of long duration shared by no others that may form the basis of affiliation extending across the life cycle. Siblings provide opportunities for bonds that are unlike any others. But the relationship is an ascribed one with little choice as to the particular participants, and some of the very factors that potentially may enrich a relationship between brothers and sisters in later life also may constrain them and cause them to sever ties. Some may choose to leave a bitter shared history behind. Even so, siblings continue to be important in the lives of many older persons.

Although relationships with siblings may wane somewhat during years of childrearing and involvement in the labor force, it is thought that barring conflicts, incompatibility, health problems, or distance, relationships may be renewed in later life (McPherson, 1983). Both gender and marital status are believed to bear on relationships with siblings. The female linkage with siblings in old age as with other interpersonal relationships and at other stages of the life cycle is stronger, with sister-sister ties frequently being more enduring than other combinations.

Although McPherson (1983) concluded that the unmarried usually maintain more ties with siblings than the married, among the unmarried it is less clear which group has the most contact with siblings. Those who fail, however, to maintain contact may be the most at risk of not having support in a crisis.

The majority of older people have siblings (three-fourths or more), and as many as one-half may have contact with them weekly (McPherson, 1983). As with other potential social ties outside the marital dyad, it has been suggested that siblings may be more significant in the lives of the childless and the unmarried. Yet siblings were not a source of sociability for a substantial minority of the unmarried men and women studied here. By time 2, 16 percent had no living siblings and another 10 to 15 percent or more depending on marital status did not interact with those they had (Table 8.1). This suggests that for almost 30 percent of these unmarried with no siblings or who had lost touch with those still remaining, brothers and sisters were unlikely to provide much informal support or care. Furthermore, there was also little exchange of financial support; few gave or received monetary assistance from siblings.

MARITAL STATUS, GENDER, AND AMOUNT OF CONTACT WITH SIBLINGS

Marital status was not associated with the number of siblings at either interview for men ($F = .46$, time 1; $F = .62$, time 2) or for women ($F = 1.29$; $F = .66$). Interaction with siblings, however, reflected marital status to a greater extent. Divorced men were more isolated from their siblings than were the never-married men both when they were younger and older ($F = 4.10$, $p < .05$, time 1; $F = 3.02$, $p < .05$, time 2). Contact with siblings by widowed men fell between that of the divorced and never married. Like never-married men, never-married women also interacted more with their siblings than did the formerly married at both times ($F = 5.49$, $p < .01$, time 1; $F = 3.55$, $p < .05$, time 2). By the end of the decade, compared to other women, the divorced were least involved with their brothers and sisters.

There were no consistent patterns of sex differences in ties with siblings within the marital status groups. For example, divorced women had more contact than divorced men with brothers and sisters at the beginning of the decade ($t = 2.80$, $p < .01$) whereas widowed women saw siblings a little more frequently than widowed men at the end of the ten-year period ($t = 1.68$, $p < .10$). And the ties of the never married with siblings were not differentiated by gender over time ($t = .98$, ns, time 1; $t = .68$, ns, time 2).

CHANGE IN CONTACT WITH SIBLINGS

Over the decade from one-quarter to one-third of the unmarried changed their pattern of affiliation with siblings (Table 8.2). In contrast to their increased association with their children, the majority who modified their patterns of affiliation with siblings withdrew from interaction. Divorced men and women and widowed men who experienced a transition in their ties with brothers and sisters especially diminished their contact with about three-fourths or more having reduced their interaction. Never-married men and women and widowed women were more likely to have increased contact than the other groups.

CORRELATES OF CHANGE IN CONTACT WITH SIBLINGS

In general, health, education, income, and employment status had little bearing on changes in relationships with siblings for most of the unmarried. Widowed men and never-married women who were retired at the beginning of the decade increased interaction with siblings in the next few years ($r = -.18$; $-.11$, respectively). Divorced men who had fared better financially decreased their ties with siblings ($r = -.11$), but never-married women with higher incomes over the decade ($r = .14$, time 1; time 2, $.22$) increased the time spent with brothers and sisters. Health at time 1 had no bearing on change for any group although widowed and divorced men in better health at the end of the decade decreased their contact with siblings ($r = -.23$; $-.15$). For most though, transitions in relationships with siblings occurred independently of social status, retirement, and health. Again, as in the instance of interaction with children there was no evidence that poor health motivated siblings to rally around one another in old age.

FRIENDSHIPS

In contrast to kinship, friendship is voluntary and permits choice. Although rates of interaction tend to be higher among relatives than that between friends, the meaningfulness of friendships exceeds that of relationships with kin (Williamson, Evans, & Munley, 1980). Time spent with friends tends to be more valued than that spent with relatives. Friendships with age peers may be more significant at some points in the life course than at others. When spouses are lost through divorce or widowhood, affiliation with one's age peers may become more frequent and more meaningful (Williamson et al., 1980).

Although siblings may die and children may be unavailable, presumably, there may be the opportunity to expand friendships in old age. As noted, reliance on children and siblings for socializing and social support does not seem to be a viable choice for a substantial proportion of the unmarried aged. In the future, the salience of friends in providing social support may be augmented if decreased rates of fertility continue, and parents perhaps have only one surviving child and no siblings. Friendships with unrelated adults might then become the major source of companionship and nurturance to single older persons (Williamson et al., 1980). Friends may be added or dropped and therefore attachments to them may be more fluid than those with kin. In the present research, it was possible to learn how interaction with friends changed and to compare it with the transitions in contact with children and siblings.

MARITAL STATUS, GENDER, AND AMOUNT OF CONTACT WITH FRIENDS

The unmarried indicated the frequency with which they phoned or saw friends face to face. Responses ranged from "Daily" through "Never." For analyses in this section, both types of contact (face-to-face and phoning) were combined.

Marital status was not associated with amount of contact with friends at time 1 among either men (F = 2.36) or women (F = .17) nor at time 2 for men (F = 1.03). But later in their lives the never married saw substantially more of their friends than did widowed or divorced women (F = 3.08, p < .05).

Gender differentiated affiliation with friends more when the unmarried were older. There were no gender differences in friendship ties for the widowed (t = 1.24) or divorced (t = 1.61) at time 1 although never-married women maintained more contact with their friends than never-married men (t = 3.47, p < .001). By the end of the decade women more than men affiliated with friends irrespective of marital status (t = 4.15, p < .001, widowed; 2.86, p < .01, divorced; 4.15, p < .001, never married). Thus never-married women over the decade successfully maintained more ties with friends than did formerly married women and never-married men.

CHANGE IN CONTACT WITH FRIENDS

Among these unmarried, relationships with friends were especially fluid compared to those with children and siblings. Men's ties with friends were most unstable with 42 to 45 percent of the widowed, divorced, and never-married men having changed their associations with friends (Table 8.2). More than 80 percent of the widowed and divorced men who experienced changes lost friends. Never-married men were a little more able to maintain friendships over time even though changes were usually decremental for them as well with 60 percent declining.

Overall women had somewhat fewer changes in friendships, but when they did have transitions, more than 70 percent experienced losses. Never-married men and women were more able to increase contact with friends than any of the other groups. Unlike the finite availability of siblings or children, contact with friends was one area in which there might have been greater opportunities for increments. Yet, there was more change in friendships than in other types of interaction and the majority of those who changed were not able to avoid losses.

CORRELATES OF CHANGE IN CONTACT WITH FRIENDS

Affiliation with friends was also more responsive to characteristics of persons' location in the social structure than were other types of interaction. Whereas changes in associations with children and siblings were largely independent of education, income, employment status, or health, transitions in ties with friends were especially responsive to education and income among women. Divorced and never-married women with more education ($r = .15; .15$) and higher incomes ($r = .14; .15$) at time 2 increased interaction with friends. Never-married men with more education ($r = .15$) also continued to enlarge their friendships over time although changes in men's affiliation with friends were less dependent on status characteristics than those of women. Furthermore, friendships tended to endure regardless of health.

RELATIONSHIPS BETWEEN CHANGES IN CONTACT

How do changes in one kind of relationship affect transitions in another? Does an increase in affiliation with one group depress that in another? For example, do persons who see their children more, in turn, reduce their time with friends? Changes in relationships in one area of life (e.g., children) were largely unrelated to those in other domains. Changes in ties with children, siblings, and friends were unrelated among women (e.g., no correlation was larger than $r = .05$). Among men statistical relationships between the various types of transitions were weak (ranging from $r = .10$ to $.16$), but they generally indicated that increases in one kind of interaction were not attained at the cost of reduction in others. If anything, increased involvement with either kin or friends seemed to encourage reaching out for other kinds of opportunities to maintain social ties. For example, increased contact with friends was accompanied by somewhat greater interaction with siblings among widowed ($r = .15$), divorced ($.13$), and never-married men ($.13$).

ISOLATION OF THE UNMARRIED

The importance of social ties for psychological well-being has long been acknowledged (Rook, 1984). Furthermore, there is also increasing interest in the linkages between social relationships and physical health as well. Evidence of the extensiveness of the social lives of older persons has been drawn from detailed social surveys assessing the range of their involvement with others. Whereas much of the research has asked persons to recount the frequency and/or amount of contact with neighbors, friends, and relatives, other efforts have tried to estimate the presence of confidants and close relationships and their importance in old age (Mouser, Powers, Keith, & Goudy, 1985).

Evidence from surveys across age groups indicates many persons lack important social bonds (Rook, 1984). One national survey, for example, found that 19 percent did not have "many very good friends" (Campbell, Converse, & Rodgers, 1976) whereas 5 percent did not know anyone to whom they could go if they had difficulties (Campbell, 1981). These findings, however, do not indicate how many had no contact with relatives and friends. Chappell (1983) found that small percentages of the elderly had *no* contact with relatives outside the home (2 percent), with close friends (1 percent), or with neighbors (2 percent). In a national study, it was found that 1 percent of persons aged 65 or over never went to the home of a neighbor or relative, and for 9 percent it had been longer than three months since they had done so (Harris & Associates, 1981). All others maintained some level of contact with relatives, friends, or neighbors. The sample, however, included the married, and availability and frequency of contact were not examined by marital status.

One way to view social ties of the unmarried is to consider those who indicate they *never* have face-to-face or phone contact with neighbors, friends, or relatives. The unmarried respondents studied here noted if they never had face-to-face contact or spoke with friends, neighbors, or relatives by telephone.

Gender was generally not linked to the absence of face-to-face contact (Table 8.3). About equal proportions of men and women never associated with neighbors and did not ever get together with friends socially (Table 8.3). Fewer were isolated from relatives, 14 percent of the women and 21 percent of the men. Thus men were a little more likely to have no face-to-face contact with relatives but

Table 8.3
Percentage Who Never Have Contact with Neighbors, Friends, and Relatives by Sex and Marital Status

	See Neighbors	Phone Neighbors	See Friends	Phone Friends	See Relatives	Phone Relatives
Marital Status			Men			
Widowed	31	59	32	45	14	18
Divorced	34	52	36	47	24	27
Never Married	36	57	22	44	24	30
Total Sample	34	56	29	45	21	26
			Women			
Widowed	32	30	31	20	12	9
Divorced	36	38	36	24	16	12
Never Married	35	31	22	19	18	15
Total Sample	33	32	30	20	14	10

they were no more isolated than women from face-to-face contact with friends and neighbors.

The major difference in the social isolation of these men and women was in contacts by telephone. For example, 20 percent of the women had no contact with friends by phone compared with 45 percent of the men who never phoned friends. There was a similar pattern of contact with neighbors and relatives by phone.

There were few consistent differences in social isolation by marital status. One pattern worth noting was that never-married men and women were least likely to be isolated from face-to-face contact with friends. Thirty-six percent of the divorced men and women, for example, never had contact with friends compared to 20 percent of the never-married men and women (Table 8.3).

Ward (1979) suggested that family members seemed to coalesce about divorced women resulting in greater family satisfaction among them than among divorced men leaving the latter especially vulnerable. These divorced men had fewer contacts in person and by phone than divorced women.

Widowers were less isolated from family than other men whereas patterns of isolation from family by the divorced more closely resembled those of never-married men. In their isolation from friends, however, divorced men were more comparable to their widowed counterparts. Clearly, disassociation from family contacts was not compensated for by increased interaction with friends by divorced men as it may have been among the never married. Although the lack of contact with friends among divorced women paralleled that of divorced men, they were not quite so isolated from family.

CORRELATES OF AMOUNT OF INFORMAL INTERACTION

Previously correlates of change in various types of interaction were considered. In this section, education, income, employment status, health, and race were examined in relation to the *amount* of contact the unmarried maintained with children, siblings, and friends. To determine whether or not different factors seemed to prompt the various types of interaction, separate multiple regressions were conducted for contact with children, siblings, and friends by marital status.

Interaction of widowed men with all types of significant others was independent of these personal characteristics. Personal characteristics had only very limited effects on the interaction of divorced and never-married men, and none of the factors consistently were associated with greater interaction across the types of social ties. Generally, by the time of the second interview, prior interaction was the most important indicator of men's participation. Among all types of interaction only friendship at time 1 failed to be the most important predictor of affiliation at time 2. As observed earlier, friendship ties of these unmarried people were the most fluid of all types of affiliation so it might be expected that earlier patterns would be poorer predictors of activity at a later time.

Among divorced men, only income had any effect on their contact with children (b = .27). Men who were better off financially were either sought out more often by their children or were more able to initiate the contact themselves. Race did not affect the frequency of interaction with children by either the widowed or divorced men. Contact with children at time 1 was the only factor significantly associated with interaction with them at time 2 among the widowed men. Personal characteristics accounted for 12 and 32 percent of the variance in interaction with children among widowed and divorced men respectively.

Whereas divorced men's contact with their children was independent of race, it figured in their contact with siblings (b = .17) and friends (b = .23) in a way it did not for other men. Divorced black men saw their brothers and sisters and friends more than their white counterparts. Enjoying better health (b = .22) also encouraged divorced men to seek out their friends, whereas only higher incomes fostered more contact of never-married men with their friends (b = .23). Background characteristics and affiliation at an earlier time explained 24, 36, and 35 percent of the variance in contact with siblings compared with 11, 19, and 11 percent for friends among widowed, divorced, and never-married men, respectively.

Women's interaction with friends was most influenced by personal characteristics. Income (b = .32) and education (b = .49) were especially important to maintaining the friendship ties of never-married women although more education (b = .22, .24), and higher income also figured significantly in maintaining friendships for the formerly married as well (b = .14, .20, widowed and divorced, respectively). These factors accounted for 17, 15, and 33 percent of the variance in contact with friends for the widowed, divorced, and never-married women. Women's interaction with friends was affected more adversely by low socioeconomic characteristics than were those of men.

Never-married women who were better off financially either sought out their siblings more frequently or were contacted by them (b = .19) although earlier contact was less important to their current interaction (b = .39) than it was for widowed (b = .49) and divorced women (b = .59). Association with siblings by widowed and divorced women was independent of social and economic factors and was largely predicted by earlier affiliation (R^2 = .24, .37, .18, widowed, divorced, never married, respectively).

LEISURE ACTIVITIES

In addition to their participation in formal organizations and with kin and friends, older people are involved in a number of other activities that may or may not include the company of friends or acquaintances. Although activities have been categorized in many ways, Robinson (1977) classified them by where they took place, for example, in the home or outside the home. In the present research, activities were considered that can be pursued in the home such as hobbies or viewing television and those undertaken outside the home, for example, going to restaurants, shopping, or attending movies, concerts, or plays. Many of the activities can be engaged in with others or participated in alone. They also vary as to cost, expenditure of energy, and need for transportation.

It was expected that frequency of engagement in activities would vary because some were accessible on a daily or more frequent basis (e.g., television or reading), whereas others were less available or perhaps selected less often (e.g., movies, plays, concerts; Table 8.4). Some research has suggested that young and old persons participate in much the same activities except for greater involvement in sports by the young and more time spent at work and activities with children and other family members (Breytspraak, 1984). Television viewing, reading, and taking walks were the most frequent activities of these older unmarried adults whereas attending movies/plays/concerts, participating in sports or exercise, and taking a trip lasting longer than a day least often occupied them.

Gender and Leisure Activities

Involvement in many of the activities was clearly gender-linked; of the ten activities, men and women participated similarly in only two— their attendance at concerts, plays, or movies and the frequency of their grocery shopping (Table 8.4). Men more often went for walks, participated in sports and exercise, and engaged in home maintenance projects. Taking walks and doing odd jobs are among the more commonly recognized masculine activities in old age (Rubinstein, 1986). These unmarried men ate more meals away from home in restaurants, perhaps reflecting less interest or skill in cooking. Women participated more frequently in activities that tend to be sedentary: viewing television, reading, working on hobbies, and taking trips.

Marital Status and Leisure Activities

The leisure activities of men were largely undifferentiated by marital status. The widowed viewed television more often ($F = 2.99$, $p < .05$), whereas the never married spent more time reading ($F = 3.94$, $p < .05$).

Leisure activities of women were more often associated with marital status; for example, widows especially engaged in more in-home pursuits. For example, widows watched television ($F = 4.68$, $p < .01$) and worked at hobbies (3.25, $p < .05$) more than never-married women. The never married participated in activities outside

Table 8.4

Mean Frequency of Involvement by Men and Women, Time 1, Time 2

	Selected Solitary and Group Activities				
	Men		Women		
Activity	Time 1	Time 2	Time 1	Time 2	t^a
Viewing Television	4.49	4.53	4.77	4.79	4.27***
Reading	4.29	4.15	4.55	4.49	4.28***
Working on Hobbies	2.42	2.28	3.18	3.13	8.70***
Shopping at Grocery	3.84	3.72	3.82	3.69	ns
Going to Restaurant	2.95	2.89	2.56	2.56	4.02***
Attending Concert/Play	1.71	1.51	1.52	1.44	ns
Taking a Trip (longer than 1 day)	2.62	1.87	2.66	2.08	3.47***
Participating in Sports/Exercise	1.52	1.39	1.29	1.26	2.27*
Taking Walks	4.15	4.07	3.57	3.55	5.80***
Home Maintenance	2.58	2.44	2.10	1.97	5.76***
	Formal Organizations				
Organization/ Club Meetings	1.57	1.57	1.92	1.92	5.94***
Church/Temple Activities	2.46	2.34	3.08	3.06	9.63***
Volunteer Work	1.23	1.16	1.46	1.46	6.89***
Senior Center (% participating)		8%		22%	

*p <.05

**p <.01

***p <.001

[a]T-Tests were used to show differences in involvement of men and women at time 2 only.

the home more than the widowed and divorced; they attended more movies, plays, and concerts ($F = 3.53$, $p < .001$) and went to restaurants more frequently ($F = 3.53$, $p < .05$). In general, however, the never married were more similar to divorced women in their participation in the ten solitary and group activities than they were to the widowed. Usually never-married women were most oriented toward activities beyond the home.

Change in Leisure Activities

To observe change in leisure activities over time, data first collected on leisure activities four years before the close of the study were compared with participation at the end of the decade (Table 8.4). As a group, these unmarried men and women changed their involvement in solitary and group activities very little over a four year period. They had increased participation in only one activity—viewing television—and then the increments were very slight. Frequency of participation declined for the remainder of the activities, but most decreases were small and tended to be similar for men and women. Although some individuals may have experienced sharp declines, as a group there was little evidence of precipitous change. These data then support other research observing consistency in activities of older persons.

SUMMARY AND DISCUSSION

Leisure that is most valued by adults of either sex and at any age involves interaction with significant others, although more actual time may be spent in other pursuits (e.g., watching television) (Kelly et al., 1986). Despite the value placed on interchanges with kin and friends, the amount of interaction often has not been found to contribute to well-being of the aged (see Lee, 1985, for a review). Unfortunately, the relative value and meaning of different kinds of interaction for these unmarried were not assessed. In a later chapter, however, analyses that consider the contribution of informal social ties and leisure activities to happiness and satisfaction with level of activity among the unmarried in urban or rural areas are reported.

When change did occur in amount of contact, it most often reflected reduced activity except for interaction with children with whom ties were increased over the decade by all but divorced men. In large part, changes in contacts were independent of social status characteristics and increased involvement in one type of interaction (for example, children and friends) was not achieved at the expense of declines in others. The relative stability in interaction with children, siblings, and friends for the majority should not obscure the finding that substantial minorities of the unmarried either had no children or brothers or sisters or did not maintain contact with those still living. Divorced men were most at risk of not having contact with children or siblings.

Like their ties with kin and friends, the involvement of these unmarried men and women in out-of-home and home-based leisure activities remained much the same over a four-year period. Some of the activities were especially gender-linked, although both men and women might have derived benefits from participation in them. In the next chapter, the relationship between these activities and well-being as well as rural-urban differences in participation are considered.

Old and Single in the City and in the Country: Activities of the Unmarried

9

THE RURAL-URBAN CONTEXT

It might be asked why we should be interested in examining some of the differences in the lives of the rural and urban aged. One reason has to do with the presumed disadvantages of the rural elderly. A considerable proportion of available gerontological research comparing the aged in urban areas with those in rural places has pointed to the disadvantaged status of the latter in income, health, housing, and transportation (Krout, 1986). Whereas the rural elderly have been described as confronting double jeopardy (i.e., old and rural), it is possible that by virtue of their marital status the unmarried in small towns and the open country may face triple risks.

A brief description of the demography of age by place of residence will establish the context in which the social relationships and activities considered in this chapter took place. More than one-quarter of the aged live in rural areas. Perhaps more important to the provision of services and programs for the aged is the proportion of an area's population that is older. In small towns in rural areas, as distinct from small communities adjacent to metropolitan regions, 15.4 percent of the population is elderly, the highest percentage for any size

Portions of this chapter originally appeared in P. Keith and A. Nauta, "Old and Single in the City and in the Country: Activities of the Unmarried." *Family Relations* 1988, 37:79–83. Used with permission of the National Council on Family Relations.

of place. The lowest percentage (10 percent) of older persons to the total population is observed in suburban or urban fringe areas (Krout, 1986). Although the dependency ratio may be larger in small rural towns that in turn may constrain the resources extended to the aged, high proportions of elderly, of course, also may translate into greater opportunities for socialization with age peers.

Generally, in contrast to males, older females are less likely to live in rural and nonmetropolitan areas. This pattern is evident in the sex ratio (i.e., the number of males per 100 females) that is 82.6 for rural areas compared with 63.0 for urban places (Bureau of the Census, 1983). Nonmetropolitan places, especially farming areas, tend to have aged populations that include a higher proportion of persons who are married (Krout, 1986). These trends are reflected in living arrangements in that except when they reside in farming areas older women are more likely than men to live alone. Thus some circumstances seem to differentiate the lives of the rural and urban elderly, and suggest that social participation, interpersonal relationships, and leisure activities also may be influenced by place of residence and vary in type and amount depending on community size.

PARTICIPATION AND ACTIVITIES OF THE RURAL AND URBAN AGED

It was recently observed that potential rural-urban differences in social relationships are crucial for older people because interaction with others has been found to be associated with various types of adjustment and emotional well-being in later life (Lee & Whitbeck, 1987). This chapter provides information on the groups and activities in which older, widowed, divorced, and never-married persons were most frequently involved in rural and urban settings. The importance of various activities to well-being and gender differences in involvement by size of place are discussed in this chapter. Findings from the research could assist practitioners in determining whether to differentiate the activities and programs they provide for rural and urban residents. Barriers to participation of the unmarried aged in both large and small communities are identified. By specifying conditions under which participation of the unmarried aged is impeded, it is possible to suggest educational and program efforts to address some of the barriers. Identification of gender-linked patterns of activity that most often promote well-being makes it possible to determine whether cross-sex leisure pursuits may warrant encouragement by those who design programs.

This research then highlights some significant issues for those who plan programs for older persons and responds to some critical questions:

1. Is there a difference between rural and urban elderly in the amount and type of activities in which they engage? If differences exist, they can be taken into account in planning strategies for intervention.

2. Are certain activities more important than others to the well-being of participants? If such activities are identified, practitioners will likely want to facilitate involvement in those which seem most beneficial.

3. To what extent do the activities and affiliation of the unmarried elderly differ from what is known about the patterns of involvement of the general aged population, which is largely based on samples of married persons? Findings from this research should aid in planning for the unmarried so that their interests are not overlooked. Until recently, affiliation and activities of both the rural and unmarried aged have been neglected.

In assessing social involvement of older persons, Kivett (1985:188) observed that "A significant void in the literature is the relative lack of research comparing the social activity of the rural to that or urban populations." Even less is known about comparative patterns of activities of the unmarried in rural and urban places. Research on affiliation and activities of the unmarried should provide useful information for practice for several reasons: (1) as observed in Chapter 1, the unmarried are a substantial and growing proportion of the aged population; (2) the older unmarried depend more on both formal and informal services than the married and therefore might be expected to benefit especially from programs designed with their social needs in mind; and (3) the unmarried are generally regarded as more vulnerable to isolation and presumably could benefit from efforts to provide opportunities for social integration (Keith, 1986).

Since clients of practitioners increasingly will be unmarried, knowledge of activities that contribute most to their well-being could be useful in deciding which programs to foster. In assessing needs and developing new programs, planners will want to take into account the extent to which activities of the unmarried and those that have positive outcomes for well-being vary by size of place.

AFFILIATION AND ACTIVITIES OF
RURAL/URBAN AGED

Comparisons of affiliation and activities of the aged in rural and urban areas often have not focused on marital status, but both the findings and some of the theories are informative. Theoretical perspectives indicating that social networks are responsive to structural opportunities and constraints suggest rival hypotheses about differences in activities of the rural and urban aged. Longstanding concern with rural-urban differences in social relationships and ideas of early writers generally led to the popular assumption that social bonds are more tenacious in rural areas and more fragmented in cities. Such conditions were thought to lead to greater social and emotional isolation in urban areas. Fischer (1982) theorized that urbanism affects the social context in which people establish their relationships with others by expanding opportunities for building ties outside the family and neighborhood. Other data, however, suggest the effects of urbanism on activities may be mitigated somewhat by the density of the aged population. Rates of interaction may be higher in communities in which the aged represent a greater proportion of the population, thus, favoring their involvement in smaller communities.

The distribution of the aged by marital status and gender in urban and rural communities also may affect their ties with others. Blau (1973) observed the adverse effect of marital status on social participation when it placed individuals in an atypical position relative to age and sex peers. In the United States, unmarried older men are not disproportionately located in either rural (22 percent) or urban areas (24 percent). Older women in urban areas, however, are somewhat more likely (65 percent) to be unmarried than their rural age peers (55 percent). Older unmarried women regardless of community size will have more same-sex, unmarried age peers with whom to affiliate.

The more varied opportunities associated with urbanism argue for greater involvement in these areas whereas concentration of the aged may increase options for interpersonal relations in rural areas. More available same-sex and age peers would favor the involvement of unmarried women over that of men regardless of location.

Although research is limited, there is some evidence that older persons in rural areas may participate less in most formal organizations than their urban counterparts (Kivett, 1985). Reasons offered for this apparent difference have included more limited personal resources of the rural aged (i.e., lower incomes, poorer health, less available transportation), fewer available options for membership, and perhaps less inclination to adopt newer opportunities for affiliation such as senior citizens' programs (Kivett, 1985). Although it might be expected that participation would thrive where there is greater density of older persons, data on this relationship have been contradictory.

Kivett (1985) concluded that in contrast to their lesser involvement in formal organizations, rural people may engage in more informal interaction with nonkin. Some of the samples, however, on which this generalization was based were limited to a particular geographical area. Other researchers have reported conflicting observations; for example, from their analyses of a number of samples, Liang and Warfel (1983) noted that objective social integration was highest among individuals living in small cities compared with persons residing in either smaller or larger places. In contrast, however, subjective integration was highest for older residents of small towns and rural areas. Still other scholars indicate that residential location has little effect on kinship ties (Lee & Whitbeck, 1987). Homogeneity in age and social class (Kivett, 1985) may favor greater informal participation in rural areas but these may be offset by more limited income and poorer transportation that especially may constrain the nonkin activities of the rural aged.

Typically kin, especially adult children, are a major source of social contact for the aged. Early research found that the urban aged more than their rural peers interacted with kin (most often children). More recent research showing greater interaction between rural families and their kin probably reflects higher rates of interaction by farmers and not of rural residents generally (Lee & Cassidy, 1985). More interaction between farmers and their children is probably due to residential proximity or joint farming operations. There is little consistent evidence that rural nonfarm families see children and other kin any more often than the aged living in larger places.

Earlier it was noted that the more limited personal resources of the rural aged may restrict their involvement with others. It has been suggested that to the degree that greater social integration characterizes the rural aged it may compensate for their striking deficits in income, health, and other factors that contribute to psychological well-being (Lee & Lassley, 1982). In this chapter, it is possible to determine the relative importance of various types of involvement and socieconomic factors for the well-being of the unmarried aged in rural and urban areas.

In addition, it was expected that factors connected to position in the social structure (education, income, employment status) and the personal resource of health would provide opportunities for formal/ informal involvement, whereas deficits in these areas would constrain participation. Good health promotes social involvement, and aspects of socioeconomic status prompt participation especially in formal organizations (Palmore, 1981).

PROCEDURES

Sample

In this chapter the unmarried were grouped by place of residence. Among the unmarried, 1,245 women, and 251 men resided in areas with populations of 2,500 or greater. In this chapter, these persons are designated as the urban sample. There were 429 women and 124 men living in communities of less than 2,500 or in the open country. These are described as the rural residents. Of the rural sample, 16 percent (n = 87) lived on farms. Because initial analyses of the variables of interest indicated that farm and nonfarm respondents were quite similar, these groups were combined. Thus comparisons were made between persons living in communities smaller than 2,500 or open country and those living in towns and cities of 2,500 or larger.

Income and Education

Income was coded into 23 categories ranging from under $1,000 to $30,000 or over. In chapter 2 it was noted that median incomes of men continued to exceed those of women at time 2 ($t = 3.63$, $p < .001$). Corresponding to other literature, rural men had significantly lower incomes and less education ($t = 2.71$, $p < .001$; $t = 3.30$, $p < .001$, respectively) than their urban counterparts. Urban women also enjoyed higher incomes ($t = 7.46$, $p < .001$) and more education ($t = 5.18$, $p < .001$) than women in small communities.

Employment Status

Employment status was coded 0 (retired), 1 (employed). Fourteen percent of the urban men and 15 percent of the rural men were employed at time 2 ($x^2 = .09$, ns). By time 2, employment was equally popular among rural and urban women ($x^2 = 00$, ns). Twelve percent of the urban women and 13 percent of the rural women remained in the labor force at time 2.

Health

Functional capacity was assessed by summing up responses to two questions: "Do you have any health condition, physical handicap, or disability that limits how well you get around?" and "Does your health limit the kind or amount of work or housework you can do?" (yes, no). A higher score indicated better health. Rural and urban men did not differ in self rated health (t = .29) whereas urban women reported somewhat better health than their counterparts in small communities (t = 2.59, p < .01).

Well-Being

Global happiness was measured by an item often used in surveys: "Taking things altogether, would you say you are happy, pretty happy, or not too happy these days?" Respondents indicated how satisfied they were with their level of activity (very unsatisfactory—more than satisfactory). Higher scores for both happiness and satisfaction with level of activity indicated more positive feelings about their lives by the unmarried.

Formal Participation

Respondents noted the number of formal organizations in which they maintained memberships. They also reported their frequency of involvement in (a) clubs and organizations; (b) church/temple activities; (c) volunteer work (not at all—daily); and (d) participation in a senior center (yes, no). Responses across the first three items which ranged from "not at all" to "daily" were summed with a higher score reflecting greater participation in formal organizations.

Informal Participation

Respondents indicated how often they had contact with siblings, relatives who were less close kin than siblings, and friends in person or by phone (daily—not at all). Contacts in person and by phone were summed with higher scores indicating higher informal participation. Preliminary analyses indicated there were no differences in contact with children by place of residence; since affiliation with children did not contribute significantly to well-being of the formerly married, interaction with children was excluded from the multivariate analyses.

Leisure Activities

Respondents reported how often they engaged in each of nine leisure activities: watching television; reading (books, magazines, newspapers); working on hobbies; doing home maintenance or small repairs; taking walks; participating in sports or exercise; going to a restaurant, cafeteria, or snackbar; going to concerts, plays, movies, and so forth; or taking a trip away from home lasting longer than one day. Responses ranged from "not at all" to "daily" with higher scores indicating greater involvement.

Analyses

T-tests and multiple regression analyses were used to address questions about rural/urban differences in participation and in the outcomes of involvement. In separate multiple regression analyses of happiness and satisfaction with level of activity, education, income, employment status, and health were always considered as the first block. In the first analysis formal/informal activities were included as the second block; in a second analysis, other leisure activities formed the second block.

RESULTS

Rural/Urban Differences in Activities

As observed in Chapter 8, television viewing, reading, and taking walks were activities that these unmarried people engaged in most frequently, and these were the most popular pastimes whether they lived in the city or in the country. Likewise, attendance at movies/plays/concerts, sports events, and volunteer work least often occupied these older unmarried adults regardless of place of residence. Of course, most of the latter activities necessitated leaving the home and for the majority of persons would be less readily available than television viewing or reading.

Table 9.1 shows both within and between sex comparisons of participation by place of residence. Results of significant t-tests are

Table 9.1
Formal/Informal and Leisure Activities by Place of Residence and Sex

Formal/Informal	Comparisons of Amount of Involvement			
	Urban Men vs. Rural Men[a]	Urban Women vs. Rural Women	Urban Women vs. Rural Men	Rural Women vs. Rural Men
Total No. of Organizations		+	+	
Clubs	+	+	+	+
Church Services		+	+	+
Volunteer Work		+	+	+
Senior Center		+	+	+
Friends	+	+	+	+
Siblings				
Relatives			+	+
Leisure Activities				
Television Viewing			+	+
Reading		+	+	+
Hobbies			+	+
Movies/Plays/Concerts	+	+		
Maintenance			-	-
Walking			-	-
Sports/Exercise	+	+	-	
Restaurant	+	+	-	-
Trips		+	+	

[a]T-tests were used to assess differences in participation by size of place and sex except a chi square analysis was used for senior center participation; signs (+, -) indicate activities on which there were significant differences. A plus (+), indicates the group mentioned first had significantly higher involvement than the second group; a minus (-) denotes significantly less involvement by the first group. (Detailed results available from author.)

indicated by a plus (+) or a minus (−) sign, The heading at the top of each column denotes the comparison group. For example, in column 1, participation of rural and urban men is compared. A plus sign opposite clubs denotes that urban men were more active in these organizations than were rural men. A minus sign would mean that the first comparison group was less involved than the second group.

When within sex comparisons were made by size of place, and significant differences in level of involvement were found, rural residents always participated less, regardless of gender (Table 9.1, cols. 1 and 2). Activities of women were more differentiated by place of residence than those of men (Table 9.1). The personal communities of urban women differed from those of men and other women. For them, urbanism seemed to have distinctive outcomes since they were most active in most types of activities—interpersonal, solitary, and in formal organizations. Their lives appeared to be fuller and more varied. Urban men and women maintained more contact with friends than their same-sex counterparts in rural areas although urban men and rural women differed little in their ties with nonkin. Rural men were most bereft of frequent contact with friends.

Perhaps the most graphic findings were the fairly consistent gender differences in activities independent of place of residence. Both rural and urban men engaged in the more traditionally gender-linked physical activities that were reported in Chapter 8. The most commonly recognized masculine activities in old age—taking walks and doing odd jobs—were dominant among these unmarried men regardless of community size. Urban men, however, were involved in exercise and sports more often than either rural men or urban women. Although urban men more often patronized restaurants than men in small towns, regardless of place of residence men depended on eating meals away from home more than women. Hobbies, volunteer work, church activities, and affiliation with relatives were more often the purview of women regardless of size of place.

To this point, rural-urban differences in participation, and distinct gender patterns in involvement have been identified. A remaining question centers around the implications of various types of participation for well-being.

Happiness

After taking personal characteristics into account, which activities were important to happiness? And were comparable activities salient to happiness among rural and urban unmarried, older people? To answer these questions, hierarchical multiple regression analyses were conducted for men and women separately in urban and rural areas. Separate analyses were completed for formal/informal activies and leisure activities (Table 9.2). Demographic characteristics were included as the initial block and were followed in the first analysis

Table 9.2
Multiple Regression Analyses of Happiness and Formal/Informal and Leisure Activities of the Unmarried in Rural/Urban Communities[a]

Personal Characteristics	Urban Men		Rural Men		Urban Women		Rural Women	
	r	Beta	r	Beta	r	Beta	r	Beta
Income[b]	.18	.14*	.19	.04	.23	.12**	.17	.04**
Education	-.03	-.06	.24	.06	.18	.06	.22	.13
Employment	.04	.08**	.08	-.02**	.07	.01**	.12	.07**
Health	.34	.30	.43	.37	.23	.17	.20	.15
R^2		.135		.220		.095		.085

Formal/Informal Activities

	r	Beta	r	Beta	r	Beta	r	Beta
Volunteer Work	.14	.16**						
Church Services	.20	.12*						
Friends					.18	.06**		
Siblings					.11	.08		
Total R^2		.192		.272		.121		.108[c]

Leisure Activities

	r	Beta	r	Beta	r	Beta	r	Beta
Hobbies	.14	.14**			.14	.06**	.14	.09*
Trips					.19	.08**		
Restaurants					.19	.08		
Sports/Exercise							-.04	-.10**
Total R^2		.171		.248[c]		.118		.114

*$p < .10$

**$p < .05$

[a]Only formal/informal and leisure activities that contributed to happiness are listed.

[b]In analyses of formal/informal and leisure activities, income, education, employment and health were included as the first block. They are shown only once.

[c]No single activity was significant at $p < .10$.

by formal/informal activities and in the second analysis by leisure pursuits.

First, place of residence made no difference in the happiness expressed by men (t = .43) and women (t = 1.37). Health contributed most to happiness regardless of residence or gender although it was most important to rural men (Table 9.2). Lower income did not diminish the happiness of rural people as it did for urban men and women. Yet, when rural women were privileged by having more education, they also were advantaged by having greater happiness.

For the most part, few of the specific formal or informal activities contributed directly to happiness, although those that were more salient should be highlighted. Involvement in volunteer work was especially important to happiness of urban men. Only urban women derived greater happiness from ties with friends and siblings. Of the leisure activities, hobbies were important to happiness among most of the respondents except for rural men. In general, the two models (formal/informal and leisure activities) were both better predictors of happiness of men, especially rural men, than of women. But this was due primarily to the strong effects of health on the happiness of rural men.

Satisfaction with Level of Activity

Similar analyses were conducted for satisfaction with level of activity as for happiness. After demographic factors were considered, formal/informal affiliations were investigated. In the next analysis, leisure activities formed the second block.

First, rural and urban men and women were equally satisfied with their levels of activity ($t = 1.56$, ns; $t = .91$, ns, men and women respectively). Across gender and place of residence, persons in good health were most satisfied with their level of activity. Of the remaining background characteristics, employment was important to satisfaction of rural women and income to urban men (Table 9.3).

No formal and informal social ties consistently contributed to satisfaction with level of activity. Urban women were more satisfied when they worked as volunteers, participated in a senior center, and belonged to a larger number of organizations. Rural men derived satisfaction from volunteer work whereas rural and urban women obtained some benefit from involvement in church activities. Urban men were more satisfied with their level of activity when they had greater involvement in activities carried out in the home, for example, hobbies, reading, and television. These were also pursuits in which men engaged less frequently than women. No single leisure activity fostered satisfaction with level of participation among all of the groups.

Table 9.3

Multiple Regression Analyses of Satisfaction with Level of Activity and Formal/Informal and Leisure Activities of the Unmarried in Rural/Urban Communities[a]

Personal Characteristics	Urban Men		Rural Men		Urban Women		Rural Women	
	r	Beta	r	Beta	r	Beta	r	Beta
Income[b]	.24	.19**	.07	.00	.17	.04	.10	.02
Education	-.06	-.12	.19	.02	.09	-.04	.09	.00*
Employment	.18	.08**	.14	.06**	.10	.05**	.15	.09**
Health	.36	.28	.35	.32	.33	.28	.25	.21
R^2	.188		.150		.122		.077	

Formal/Informal Activities

	r	Beta	r	Beta	r	Beta	r	Beta
Volunteer Work			.25	.19*	.19	.08**		
No. of Organizations					.17	.08**		
Senior Center					.15	.07*		
Church Services					.17	.05	.14	.09*
R^2	.228		.212		.169		.100	

Leisure Activities

	r	Beta	r	Beta	r	Beta	r	Beta
Reading	.25	.16**					.16	.10*
Hobbies	.22	.15**			.16	.11**		
TV Viewing	.19	.14						
Walking							.12	.10**
Restaurant					.15	.07**		
Trips					.16	.05		
R^2	.30		.200[c]		.147		.104	

* $p < .10$

** $p < .05$

[a]Only formal/informal and leisure activities that contributed to happiness are listed.

[b]In analyses of formal/informal and leisure activities, income, education, employment and health were included as the first block. They are shown only once.

[c]No single activity was significant at $p < .10$.

Formal/Informal Participation

Lower income constrained the involvement of all men and women in formal organizations. Income tended to have a weaker influence on informal ties although low income was a barrier to maintaining relationships with kin and friends as well as memberships in formal organizations (Table 9.4). Education facilitated the involvement of both groups of women in formal organizations, and it fostered more informal ties by rural women as well. Although the models generally explained little variance, they tended to be somewhat more efficient predictors of formal than informal activities, especially those of rural men for whom both income and employment particularly increased their opportunities to participate in formal organizations. Thus some of the resources in which rural residents often tend to be disadvantaged (e.g., income, education) were important to the integration of these unmarried aged into their communities. As observed above, however, somewhat fewer formal and informal activities encouraged

Table 9.4
Multiple Regression Analyses of Formal/Informal Activities and Personal Characteristics of the Unmarried in Rural/Urban Communities[a]

Personal Characteristics	Formal Activities							
	Urban Men		Rural Men		Urban Women		Rural Women	
	r	Beta	r	Beta	r	Beta	r	Beta
Income	.20	.20**[a]	.35	.28**	.26	.15**	.28	.17**
Education	.08	--	.24	.09**	.26	.16	.28	.18*
Employment	.02	--	.26	.21	.02	-.04**	.15	.09**
Health	.04	.01	.18	.12	.20	.16	.17	.10
R^2		.040		.197		.112		.128
	Informal Activities							
Income	.14	.16**	.24	.21**	.19	.16**	.16	.09***
Education	-.01	-.04	.14	.04	.12	.03	.17	.12
Employment	--	--**	.06	.02*	.04	-.01**	.10	.08
Health	.22	.20**	.18	.15	.11	.08	.08	.04
R^2		.066		.085		.042		.046

* $p < .10$

** $p < .05$

[a] Variables (--) did not enter the equation.

happiness among rural people compared to those from urban areas. Additionally, except for volunteer work for rural men and church activities for women, formal/informal participation had little significance for satisfaction of these rural residents.

SUMMARY AND IMPLICATIONS FOR PRACTICE

Did these data suggest that practitioners may want to distinguish between rural and urban aged as they plan programs and activities? In general, urban women manifested the most diverse participation and rural men the least. Assuming that frequent associations and contacts would translate into social support when needed, then urban women were indeed the most favored and rural men the least. Urban women capitalized on the diversity of an urban environment in ways that urban men did not although their comparatively more peripatetic involvement was not reflected in greater satisfaction with level of activity.

Health was especially critical to the well-being of unmarried rural men who may have relied more on physical labor to sustain themselves, particularly those living on farms. These men had comparatively tenuous connections with their communities and should their health become precarious they would seem even more vulnerable. Frail, unmarried rural men especially may warrant the attention of practitioners.

Effects of size of place and gender tended to blur for urban men and rural women. Urban men probably benefited some from the greater offerings of their communities, whereas perhaps gender-linked interests and sociability more characteristic of females enabled women in rural areas to compensate for some of the limitations of their environment. Other research points to the need for educational and intervention programs to take into account differences in resources among categories of the unmarried, for example, widowed, divorced (Hennon, 1983).

Were activities in which persons participated less than their peers those which contributed to well-being? Volunteer work, for example, was an activity that brought urban men happiness and provided satisfaction for rural men. Indeed, volunteer work seemed to perform a function for men that it did not for rural women. But earlier analyses showed that men were also less likely to participate. In instances, volunteering may have been a meaningful extension of a former work environment for men. Although volunteer work may be a form of leisure activity for the employed, some retired clearly regard it as work. For example, only 3 percent of a sample of retirees agreed that volunteer work was a leisure activity. In contrast, 13 percent specifically identified volunteer activities as work (Roadburg, 1981). Furthermore, it is an activity that practitioners may want to encourage and for which a need exists.

Although volunteer work was particularly satisfying to rural men, structured opportunities to volunteer may be less prevalent in these areas. Such activities might help men especially if they were to capitalize on their interests and skills in maintenance and small repairs. Practitioners may want to ensure that opportunities to volunteer are available and that special efforts are made to extend them to men.

The activities in which men were more involved than women were not those most important to their happiness or satisfaction. Urban men, for example, were more satisfied with their level of activity when they had greater involvement in activities in which women participated more, for example, hobbies, reading, television. Except for health, hobbies were the most consistent source of well-being across gender and size of place. Increased encouragement of hobbies may be especially useful for older urban men. A point can be made about the location of activities that contribute most to happiness. Leisure activities bringing the most happiness more often were those taking place outside the home. Of the in-home pastimes, only hobbies, not television viewing or reading, brought some happiness.

Although eating out was not associated with well-being for men, it was a frequent activity and may, in part, have reflected the limited cooking skills of single men. Neighborhood and small town restaurants are also places for socializing on a fairly regular basis. The frequency with which single men ate away from home suggests that nutrition education should be a component of programming for older singles. It may be especially difficult for older people to adhere to prescribed diets when eating in restaurants.

Senior centers are often among the most visible organizations for the aged although involvement in them per se was not directly important to happiness or satisfaction of these single men and women. Yet, they would seem to be ideal places to foster some of the activities and skills that contributed to well-being.

Were rural men and women disadvantaged by having less income and education? When rural people had lower incomes, their happiness was not diminished as it was for urban residents. Although low income constrained participation in formal and informal activities of both men and women regardless of size of community, the effects of finances were strongest for the involvement of rural men. Rural women were advantaged when they had more education thereby enjoying greater happiness. Education may have provided rural women with competencies and skills that gave them a boost to overcome some of the other barriers to participation in smaller communities.

Education may have also enhanced the employment opportunities of older women. Continued employment, perhaps reflecting their less adequate incomes, was important to rural men and women in ways it was not for urban residents. Employment facilitated participation of rural men and women in formal activities, and it contributed to the satisfaction of rural women as well. Although opportunities for employment in small communities are dwindling, this research indicated its importance to older, unmarried rural men and women.

To what extent did these findings for older singles mirror other conclusions on rural/urban differences in participation by the aged? First, it should be made clear that little research has been conducted that permits rural/urban comparisons, and residence is not often considered in studies of leisure and recreation (Krout, 1986). Krout (1986) speculated that given the lack of public transportation and fewer services available, there might be lower rates of participation in formal leisure activities in rural areas. Furthermore, it has been suggested that church activities may be particularly important to the rural aged. Krout (1986:58) also allowed that "Solitary leisure pursuits or simple visiting of friends could also be expected to be more frequent among the rural elderly."

The "simple" pleasures of visiting friends, solitary leisure pursuits, or church involvement were not found to occupy these rural men and women more than their urban counterparts. For example, integration into religious activities was not a greater part of the lives of these rural people. In fact, urban women were most involved whereas male participation in church activities was not differentiated by place of residence. And urban men and women seemed to cultivate more ties with friends than did their age peers in the country. Therefore, homely joys, perhaps reflected in more friends, advantages often attributed to rural life and that would seem to be available despite community structural deficits, were not observed in greater abundance for these unmarried aged living in small towns or open country.

It should be pointed out that although systematic research comparing friend and neighbor ties in rural/urban communities is sketchy, most have tended to find that these informal ties favor rural residents.

Clearly, findings for these unmarried men and women fail to support this previous work. Of course, there may be several reasons for this; much previous research has not used national samples and has been region-specific if not based on a single community. The variability of the rural aged population and the differing community structural characteristics that would be excluded in a limited geographical sample might obscure differences that extend beyond a region. Finally, the findings may indicate that community size has different implications for the unmarried.

Perhaps most important, the findings underscored that the influence of size of place was tempered primarily by gender. All urban people were not more involved in formal organizations, as suggested by some research; for example, urban men were not usually more active than rural women. Women embraced the diversity of urbanism more than men, In contrast to some findings (Kivett, 1985), rural life did not result in a greater abundance of ties with nonkin. And affiliation with family (siblings, other relatives) reflected gender more than place.

Variation in patterns of participation by gender may reflect differential socialization, divergent personality characteristics, greater sensitivity and interest in other people by women, and selection of women with more social skills into urban areas combined with community structural characteristics that may have favored women in the city. It was not possible to ferret out how much of the difference in affiliation and activities of rural and urban people was due to structural effects of similarity (e.g., sex, marital status, age) of available peers versus that attributable to greater opportunities for participation in larger places. Even so, these data suggested that educational and intervention efforts should not ignore place of residence and gender.

Finally, on meager measures of well-being, quality of life did not seem to vary much by size of place. But variation in the style of life and the content of the days of these old unmarried people suggested that much of importance was probably left uncaptured.

Vulnerability of the Unmarried   **10**

INTRODUCTION

Vulnerability of the aged is a prevalent theme in popular literature as well as in writings on social gerontology. In this chapter I consider some of the personal and social situations that are thought to make the elderly especially assailable by negative life events. Although vulnerability is a common feature of much writing that depicts what it is like to be old, the connection between the life circumstances that presumably increase the risk of the aged to various unfortunate events and the actual occurrence of them is often unclearly specified.

The aged are viewed as vulnerable on a number of counts. And perhaps being unmarried is conceived of as a preeminent marker of vulnerability to a diminished quality of life in old age. When the absence of an intimate relationship is thought to be linked with loneliness, such a circumstance especially is construed as problematic. Furthermore, vicissitudes of income, health, and group memberships of the unmarried also are portrayed as enhancing vulnerability and fostering deficits particularly when compared to these characteristics among the married. Whereas some persons may have been victimized by poor health and poverty and relegated to marginal positions throughout their lives, physical aging may undermine at least a portion of their remaining resources. For some, the balance of their resources may not be enough to maintain independence. Thus aging may augment conditions of lifelong marginality and/or introduce new circumstances that increase exposure to and opportunity for even greater fragility. This is a dominant view. Nevertheless, some individuals are not overwhelmed and buffeted by situations that to others might seem to presage dwindling opportunities for physical and mental well-being in old age. In this chapter, I consider four sets of circumstances that are sometimes thought to increase the vulnerability of older persons to a poorer quality of life. These are social isolation, living arrangements, consequences of homemaking versus employment for women, and childlessness.

In the first section of this chapter, patterns of isolation/satisfaction are studied in relation to social and personal resources. Several questions may be asked about the outcomes of social isolation. Are the consequences of social isolation usually negative? What are the effects of positive or negative assessments of limited social ties? How do personal resources differentiate patterns of isolation/satisfaction?

Living arrangements of the unmarried are addressed in the second section. Frequently living arrangements are profiled as placing persons at risk of isolation and increased vulnerability to often unstated difficulties believed to be associated with living alone. In addition to other unspecified negative outcomes thought to characterize living alone, it is often viewed as a corollary of loneliness in old age. Thus although it is taken as a marker of independence and can give a sense of control over one's life, living alone also is seen as contributing to heightened vulnerability to social isolation. Questions raised in section two are: "How were living arrangements of the unmarried differentiated by marital status? Were these never married more likely to be living alone than the widowed and divorced? Were there gender differences in living arrangements?" In this section it was possible to compare well-being among the unmarried who lived alone, those who lived with others as heads of households, and those living with others as nonheads of households.

In the third section, the influence of employment decisions, some of which were made much earlier in the life course, on financial and psychological well-being are considered. There has been much debate in the literature about the outcomes of employment for women both in youth and later in life. The connection of employment with the general issue of vulnerability is usually phrased in terms of which groups (employed, retired, or homemakers) are at greater risk of poor adjustment in their later years. Often comparisons have been drawn between women who continue to work in old age, those who have been employed but have retired, and those who have been homemakers throughout their lives. The issue of which groups are more vulnerable to poorer adaptation in old age frequently has been couched with reference to the effects of employment on social relationships, finances, and psychological well-being. In this chapter, three different patterns of employment were considered in relation to finances, satisfaction with level of activity, and happiness.

The final topic involves an examination of the consequences of being a parent in comparison with having no children for the formerly married. Since the unmarried draw on the resources of children more than those living with spouses, the absence of children may be especially critical to them.

PART I: PATTERNS OF ISOLATION/SATISFACTION

Considerable study of the potential functions of close interpersonal relationships for both physical and mental health (Rook, 1984) has suggested the importance of social ties in mitigating some of the otherwise negative effects of unpleasant and often unexpected life events. In general, social isolation has been regarded as a deficit (Perlman & Peplau, 1984). And some research indicates that isolates are more apt to be lonely, have poorer morale, and generally have less positive assessments of life (see Perlman & Peplau, 1984, for a review) as well as higher rates of mortality due to alcoholism and suicide (Hughes & Gove, 1981). Lending credence to its negative image, at a World Experts on Aging Conference held at the United Nations, isolation was viewed as bad in and of itself and not just because of its consequences, which are not well established (Bennett, 1980). "Like illness, it is regarded by experts as a problem that must be solved, or perhaps as a social defect" (Bennett, 1980:3). As indicated in Chapter 1, at various times in history, singleness has also been viewed as a social defect, whereas in both popular and scientific writing isolation has been presented as a probable corollary of nonmarriage.

But negative outcomes do not always follow from isolation, and not all older persons are disadvantaged by spending much of their lives without the company of others. Some persons may intentionally cultivate privacy or embrace freedom that being alone may bring. They may be alone but not lonely (Gubrium, 1975). Not only does this suggest some potential benefits of isolation but also that isolation may reflect choice. Rather, what may be problematic is the mismatch between persons' social relationships and their needs and preferences for interaction (Perlman & Peplau, 1984). This assumes that individuals maintain preferences for amounts of interaction and that they actively evaluate those which they have (e.g., amount and quality). A cognitive discrepancy approach to isolation-interaction theorizes that persons make assessments of their relationships based on subjective standards that have origins in past relationships and/or social comparisons (Janigian, Paloutzian, & Thompson, 1986).

There are at least four patterns that close relationships and their assessment may take. The literature suggests we would find that the majority of persons desire social ties, maintain a number that is pleasing to them, and thrive on these relationships. These persons may be described as the satisfied affiliated. However, since some persons are apparently gratified by minimal contact with others, we could expect to find individuals who have few social ties but who define them positively and/or desire no more. These individuals are referred to as satiated isolates. In contrast, desolate isolates also may have few ties but feel they are deficient in interpersonal stimulation and prefer more contact. Finally, the dissatisfied affiliated maintain contact with others but desire an even greater level of activity. This chapter does not address the situation in which persons may desire to maintain fewer ties with others, perhaps reflecting interaction overload. Depending on the circumstances, if such a preference is acted on, it may be described as withdrawal.

In this portion of the chapter, I compare characteristics of unmarried men and women in relation to the four patterns of isolation/satisfaction. This analysis addresses the question of "what aspects of the lives of unmarried men and women differentiate patterns of isolation/satisfaction?" Since the relationships of desolate isolates and the dissatisfied affiliated reflect a mismatch between their preferences and their ties with others, it was anticipated that personal and social characteristics would differentiate them from individuals who were able to articulate desired and actual interaction more to their liking. To the degree that personal resources (e.g., health, income, employment) may affect social skills, enhance opportunities for forming ties with others, and promote physical mobility, it was expected that persons less able to minimize discrepancies between preferences for affiliation and actual interaction would be more disadvantaged in terms of these resources. It was anticipated that persons with disparate preferences and attainments of social ties would enjoy less happiness. More specifically, it was expected that the desolate isolates and the dissatisfied affiliated would have poorer physical health, lower income, and be less happy than persons with fewer inconsistencies in their relationships.

PROCEDURES

Typology of Isolation/Satisfaction

A typology of isolation and the response to isolation was derived by cross-classifying amount of contact with children, siblings, relatives (less close kin than siblings), and friends by satisfaction with level of activity. Persons who reported contact with children, siblings, relatives, and friends ranging from "at least monthly" to "never" were designated as more isolated whereas individuals with more frequent association (daily, weekly) were categorized as not isolated. These categories of isolated-not isolated formed one portion of the typology. To construct the part of the typology based on persons' evaluations of their level of activity, reports of satisfaction with activity ranging from "very dissatisfied" to "very satisfied" were used. The four response categories were dichotomized into satisfied/dissatisfied. Four patterns of reactions to social ties resulted from cross-classifying isolation (isolated/not isolated) by satisfaction/dissatisfaction: (1) desolate isolates (isolated, dissatisfied); (2) satiated isolates (isolated, satisfied); (3) dissatisfied affiliated (not isolated; dissatisfied); (4) satisfied affiliated (not isolated; satisfied).

Analyses

Separate analyses were conducted for the men and women. One-way analyses of variance were used to assess the bivariate relationships between the four patterns of isolation/satisfaction and personal characteristics (income, education, physical health, employment status, and happiness). Discriminant analyses were employed to examine all personal characteristics simultaneously in relation to the four patterns in a multivariate model. The intent was to present descriptive profiles of the four types rather than to assess the causal ordering of the variables.

RESULTS

As expected, the majority of the unmarried were satisfied affiliated (70 percent). Twenty percent, however, were dissatisfied affiliated who despite having a number of associates desired even more. Of the isolates, more were content with their relatively infrequent affiliation with others (7 percent) than not (4 percent desolate isolates). Although most persons had been able to attain congruence between their preferences and activities, factors that would differentiate between the patterns were of primary interest in this chapter. That is, were there personal and social resources that characterized individuals whose preferences and activities were consonant in contrast to those who experienced dissonance?

There was a significant relationship between sex and patterns of isolation/satisfaction (Table 10.1). Men were more often desolate

Table 10.1
Patterns of Isolation/Satisfaction by Marital Status (Percentages)

Patterns of Isolation/Satisfaction	Men Widowed	Divorced	Never Married	Total
Desolate Isolates	5	10	6	7
Satiated Isolates	11	12	14	12
Dissatisfied Affiliated	18	20	17	19
Satisfied Affiliated	66	58	63	62

$x^2 = 4.03$, 6 df, ns

Patterns of Isolation/Satisfaction	Women Widowed	Divorced	Never Married	Total
Desolate Isolates	2	6	3	3
Satiated Isolates	5	6	10	6
Dissatisfied Affiliated	20	26	15	20
Satisfied Affiliated	73	63	72	71

$x^2 = 28.35$, 6 df, p<.001

Total $x^2 = 35.19$, 3 df, p<.001

(7 percent) or satiated isolates (12 percent) than were women (3 percent, 6 percent, desolate and satiated isolates, respectively) who tended to be satisfied and affiliated (71 percent) to a somewhat greater extent than men (62 percent).

Marital status was associated with patterns of isolation/satisfaction among women but not among men (Table 10.1). Divorced women were more often in patterns in which preferences and attainments were incongruent and were left wanting more. Divorced women were more frequently desolate isolates, but when they were affiliated, they were somewhat more dissatisfied as well. The never married were twice as often contented and isolated as were the widowed.

It was anticipated that desolate isolates and the dissatisfied affiliated would have more negative circumstances than those who were satisfied with their social ties regardless of their isolation. One-way analyses of variance indicated that among men, the polar types, that is, the desolate isolates and the satisfied affiliated differed from one another on health ($F = 19.52$, $p < .001$) and happiness ($F = 29.45$, $p < .001$) with the desolate isolates being the most disadvantaged. Isolation per se was not a critical determinant of happiness because satiated isolates were happier than desolate isolates and the dissatisfied affiliated and enjoyed happiness comparable to that of the satisfied affiliated. Income and education of men were not significantly related to their patterns of isolation/satisfaction ($F = 1.38$; 1.13) although the satiated isolates and satisfied affiliated tended to have the highest incomes (9.33, 9.29, income category) followed by the dissatisfied affiliated (8.48) and desolate isolates (7.80).

Among women, health ($F = 62.23$, $p < .001$), income ($F = 16.95$, $p < .001$), education ($F = 4.60$, $p < .01$), and happiness ($F = 71.09$, $p < .001$) were related to patterns of isolation/satisfaction. The polar types of desolate isolates and satisfied affiliated were differentiated on all but education. The satiated isolates had the lowest educational level of any pattern. Women, however, who were content with their isolation had better health and were happier than women who had many contacts but wanted more. Women who were comfortable with their isolation were as happy as the satisfied affiliated despite their somewhat poorer health, lower incomes, and more limited education.

Multivariate Analyses of Isolation/Satisfaction

Two models of patterns of isolation/satisfaction were considered using discriminant analyses. In the first model, education, income,

Table 10.2

Discriminant Analyses of Patterns of Isolation/Satisfaction for Unmarried Men and Women: Standardized Discriminant Function Coefficients

	Men		Women			
	Model I[a]	Model II	Model I		Model II	
	Function 1	Function 1	Function 1	Function 2	Function 1	Function 2
Education	-.26	-.14	-.14	.32	-.20	.31
Income	.17	.06	.30	.78	-.13	.80
Health, Time 2	.92	.50	.88	-.40	.59	-.02
Employment Status	.16	.15	.19	.05	.13	.13
Happiness	——	.71	——	——	.69	-.35
x^2	67.05, 12 df, p<.001	113.72, 15 df p<.001	216.90, 12 df, p<.001	20.68, 6 df, p<.01	351.85, 15 df, p<.001	26.57, 8df, p<.001
Canonical Correlation	.40	.51	.34	.11	.43	.12

[a] Only function 1 is presented for men since additional functions were not significant

health, and employment status were investigated in relation to isolation/satisfaction. The second model differed in that happiness was also included. Separate analyses were conducted for men and women (Table 10.2). In the discriminant analysis of isolation/satisfaction patterns for men, there was only one significant function indicating that health differentiated the satisfied affiliated from the other three groups (Table 10.2). In the second model in which happiness was included, there was again one significant function. Although health was still an important discriminator, happiness was stronger, and both differentiated the satisfied affiliated from other patterns. In each of the analyses, however, the satiated isolates were located closest to the satisfied affiliated.

In analyses for women, there were two significant functions in the first model. As for men, health primarily differentiated between the satisfied affiliated and others. In the second function, although a less important one, income distinguished between the isolated and the nonisolated. When happiness was included in the model, there were again two significant functions. The desolate isolates and the dissatisfied affiliated were differentiated from the satiated isolates and satisfied affiliated by happiness. Thus among women happiness discriminated between those whose preferences for interaction and their social relationships were mismatched and those whose desires for affiliation and level of activity were consonant.

SUMMARY AND DISCUSSION

Being unmarried and not having close interpersonal ties are both viewed as problematic in the popular press and in much social science literature. This research permitted a limited test of whether isolation per se was linked to negative circumstances or whether isolation was disadvantageous primarily when relationships were discrepant with desires for affiliation.

First, these findings questioned the perspectives that promulgate minimal social contacts as deficits at least from the viewpoint of isolates. Although most persons were not isolated, the majority of isolates (66 percent) were satisfied with their level of activity. For both men and women, the most positive situation generally was to be satisfied and affiliated and the most negative to be isolated and want more contact with others. Having to manage discrepancies between preferred and actual ties, however, seemed more problematic than isolation per se.

The desolate isolates and dissatisfied affiliated who were both confronted with discrepancies between what they had and what they wanted usually closely resembled one another in personal resources and were among the unhappiest people. Although the dissatisfied affiliated apparently were able to maintain an array of interpersonal contacts, they remained disconsolate about the amount of activity.

Happiness was the most salient of all personal characteristics in differentiating between patterns of isolation/satisfaction of both men and women. The multivariate analysis indicated that happiness most clearly differentiated women with mismatched preferences and activities from those whose desires and attainments were more balanced, independent of their isolation. But patterns of isolation/satisfaction of both men and women also were responsive to health with the satisfied affiliated enjoying the best health.

Although the satisfied affiliated usually were the most advantaged, isolation alone did not ensure a life characterized by discontent nor did more social ties guarantee positive outlooks on life. Being isolated and satisfied was as conducive to happiness as being more engaged with others and assessing activities favorably. Even though women who were satiated isolates had very low incomes and poorer health than the satisfied affiliated, they were able to come to terms with these deficits and nourished happiness equal to that of the former. Consequently, those who work with the isolated will want to learn how isolation is evaluated because isolation alone should not be used to target persons who may be most in need of assistance. Rather isolation and preferences should be entertained together. Although most of these older unmarried persons were not isolated, a substantial proportion of those who were did not find it a desolate experience.

PART II: LIVING ARRANGEMENTS OF THE UNMARRIED

As is noted in the previous section, living alone is often seen as a marker of isolation and potential loneliness. Yet, increasingly the aged live by themselves and living alone is a more dominant pattern as persons age. For example, between the ages of 65 and 74, 34 percent of women and 11 percent of men live alone; following age 75, however, these percentages increase to 45 and 19 percent of women and men, respectively (Hess, 1985). The most marked change over time has occurred for women. From 1965 to 1981, the proportions living with other relatives declined from 19 to 10 percent with a parallel increase during the same time period in the proportion who lived alone, from 31 to 40 percent. These striking changes have been possible because of women's increased income, their ability to manage independent housing, in large part due to improved Social Security Benefits, and changing norms. Instead of living with family members, which was a more common practice earlier, women now opt to live alone. And a high value is placed on independent living.

In this section, I consider factors associated with types of living arrangements used by these unmarried men and women at the beginning and end of the decade. But first, other research on personal characteristics associated with living arrangements as well as outcomes of decisions about where to live are considered.

LIVING ARRANGEMENTS IN OLD AGE

Rubinstein (1985) identified three areas of concern that gerontologists and others have investigated in relation to living alone, but the considerations also would apply to any living arrangements. These are:

1. Factors antecedent to the living arrangement (e.g., fertility, gender, marital status, ethnic and cultural values). These factors may figure in the decision by the aged to choose a particular living arrangement (Clifford et al., 1981-82; Fillenbaum & Wallman, 1984; Glick, 1979; Soldo et al., 1984; Thomas & Wister, 1984). Research of this type primarily has considered demographic characteristics that affect decisions about living arrangements.

2. A second kind of investigation has explored social correlates of various living arrangements, that is, the events and experiences that are, in part, determined by the particular living conditions themselves. These studies may examine the social support provided by living arrangements. Rubinstein suggests that we know very little about the daily experiences of living alone in old age, but we probably know equally little, for example, about being an unmarried head of a household or living as a nonhead of a household with others in later life.

3. A third area of examination has focused on the specific outcomes and consequences of living arrangements for the elderly or their families (Arling, 1976; Mindel, 1979; Mindel & Wright, 1982a, 1982b; Fengler et al., 1983; Lawton et al., 1984; O'Bryant, 1985; and Davis et al., 1985). In these studies both objective and subjective outcomes, the latter of which are often defined as life satisfaction or morale, are considered.

FACTORS IN THE CHOICE OF LIVING ARRANGEMENTS

Perhaps marital status affects living arrangements the most. Glick (1979) observed that the most typical living arrangement for an individual in his/her late 60s was being married and living with the spouse. Fillenbaum and Wallman (1984:348) found that "married couples almost invariably lived together." Less than 2 percent of the husbands and wives lived apart. By the time persons were 85 years old and over they were less likely to be living with a spouse (Glick, 1979). By age 85, about one-third of men still resided with a spouse, whereas only 8 percent of women continued to live with a marriage partner. With increased age and change in marital status older individuals usually have transitions in living arrangements as well. Lawton (1981) noted that most people age 65 and over who were not presently married (i.e., divorced, widowed, never married) lived alone. The remainder lived with relatives or with unrelated individuals.

A second factor that influences choice of living arrangement is the level of dependency of the elderly person (Clifford et al., 1981–82). Those who must have needs met by others more likely will be found in living arrangements with other person(s), whereas the less dependent can choose to live alone. Clifford et al. (1981–82) observed that dependency had an effect on the choice of where to live as well, because those who were in living arrangements where they relied more on others experienced greater residential mobility than those who were independent. Persons who live with others because of dependency may be forced to relocate with their caregivers.

Soldo et al. (1984) examined data from 1976 Survey of Income and Education to determine the effects of age, marital status, personal income, and need for functional assistance on older unmarried women's choice of living arrangements. They found that all of these factors, with the exception of marital status, had a significant effect on the selection of living arrangements. Those in the highest income group were four times more likely to live alone than those in the lowest income group. And using their best-fitting model, they concluded that an unimpaired older woman was seven times more likely to live alone than a woman who needed assistance. Thus poor health may prompt choices of living arrangements; however, as is observed below, health practices also may be adopted in response to the living arrangements of individuals.

Thomas and Wister (1984) examined the effect of ethnicity on living arrangements of older, formerly married women and included such factors as age, education, fertility, and income. In two separate analyses with British/French and Jewish/Italian ethnicity dichotomized, fertility was the most important determinant and ethnicity the second most salient factor in the selection of living arrangements.

Thus they concluded that women who had more children were more likely to reside with one of those children. In addition, they attributed differences by ethnicity to subcultural norms that made French and Italian widows more likely to live with children than their British and Jewish counterparts.

THE CONSEQUENCES OF LIVING ARRANGEMENTS

Similarly, studies of how particular living arrangements affect the elderly and their families have been diverse. Mindel and Wright (1982a) investigated the satisfaction of primary caregivers who were living in multigenerational households. In this research, the satisfaction of older individuals was not considered, but the results of the study have important implications for the well-being of the aged also. Specifically, it was found that lower satisfaction on the part of the caregiver was associated with greater dependency of the elderly person for whom they cared. The fact that level of dependency is important in determining living arrangements, combined with the depressing effect of dependency on the well-being of caregivers, may mean that large numbers of those who provide assistance in multigenerational households will be dissatisfied.

In another study, Mindel and Wright (1982b) also examined how certain living arrangements affected the morale and subjective well-being of the elderly. After controlling for race, sex, socioeconomic status, and health, they concluded that living arrangement was a significant predictor of morale. Elderly living with a spouse had the highest level of morale, the aged living with children the lowest morale, and elderly living alone were in between. They attributed this to a negative attitude toward sharing a household with adult children. Although living arrangements did affect morale, they did not influence some other measures of subjective well-being.

Lawton et al. (1984) examined the relationship between marital status and living arrangements and the subsequent effects of the latter on various indicators of well-being (both objective and subjective). Presently married elderly were in the most favorable situation, regardless of living arrangement. Among those no longer married or never married, living alone was associated with lower subjective well-being whereas those living with children showed both lower basic competence and lower subjective well-being.

Fengler et al. (1983) also examined the effects of three types of living arrangements: living alone, living with others, and living with a spouse. They concluded that elderly people living with others were not significantly different from married couples in general life satisfaction. Widows living alone more often had low life satisfaction. The researchers attributed this to such factors as not owning their homes, perceived inadequacy of income, lack of transportation, and a fear that no one would take care of them in an emergency.

It is thought that social support from family, friends, and neighbors contributes to morale and objective needs of the aged and that it is necessary to living alone successfully (Arling, 1976; O'Bryant, 1985). O'Bryant (1985) noted that this was especially applicable to recent widows who may have depended on their husbands to handle many of the family's affairs, although neighbors and friends were more important to the morale of widows than family (Arling, 1976). Arling maintained that this was due to the voluntary nature of such relationships and the emphasis on mutual exchange of assistance. Family relationships are more likely a consequence of obligation and may result in dependency.

In research on an objective assessment of the outcome of living arrangements, Davis et al. (1985) examined dietary patterns of 3,477 adults aged 65 to 74. Contrasting results were found for men and women. Living with a spouse was associated with a more favorable dietary pattern than living alone among men. Low-income men who lived alone were at the highest risk of poor dietary intake. Living arrangements were not as important predictors of diet as was income for women. Women below the poverty level exhibited poorer dietary intake regardless of their type of living arrangement.

It is clear that marital statuses provide a range of emotional and physical support that in turn shape health outcomes. But living arrangements also may figure in decisions to seek physician care, use hospitals, or in daily health maintenance activities. Wolinsky and Coe (1984) observed that the effect of living alone was twice as important as the influence of being married or widowed on use of physician services. Other research has concurred in finding that persons living alone were more likely to consult physicians and had a larger number of visits during the year than individuals living with others (Cafferata, 1984). Whereas those living alone may use more health services, they also tend to report having better health (Tissue & McCoy, 1981), fewer functional disabilities, and fewer or no limitations in daily activities (Lawton et al., 1984) than those in other living arrangements. Irrespective of marital status, those who lived with others had more bed disability days, but they had fewer physician visits, suggesting that others in the household may provide substitute services in lieu of the use of the formal health care system (Cafferata, 1987).

A common thread through much of this research is that elders who are married fare best perhaps as a consequence of both their living arrangements and marital status. Even so, most of the unmarried live alone in their old age. In the sections that follow factors that were linked with living arrangements of these unmarried men and women are considered.

LIVING ARRANGEMENTS OF UNMARRIED
MEN AND WOMEN OVER TIME

Because household composition was coded somewhat differently at the two interviews, it was necessary to derive a set of common categories to assess change in living arrangements over the decade. At time 1, the following categories of living arrangements were included: (a) the respondent alone; (b) the respondent with children, or with children and other relatives; (c) with other relatives; (d) with nonrelatives and others. At the later interview, more specific additional groupings were used to determine the relationship of the respondent to the head of the household. It was possible to determine if the unmarried were living not only with children, but also with parents, grandchildren, in-laws, stepparents, or siblings.

Bernard (1972) observed that whether or not persons were heads of households seemed to have differential significance for the psychological well-being of males and females. To take this into account, in this research, I categorized respondents' status as head of a household and their household composition at times 1 and 2 in the following ways: (1) heads of households living alone; (2) heads of households living with others; and (3) nonheads of households living with others.

RESULTS

The living arrangements of these unmarried men and women reflected national trends since those living alone increased as they aged over the decade. At the time of the first interview 55 percent of the respondents were heads of households and were living alone, whereas by time 2, over two-thirds (68 percent) were living alone (Table 10.3). The proportion of respondents who were heads of households but living with others declined from one-third at time 1

Table 10.3
Living Arrangements by Sex and Marital Status at Time 1 and Time 2
(Percentages)

	Men					
	HH, alone		HH, others		Non H, Others	
	Time 1	Time 2	Time 1	Time 2	Time 1	Time 2
Widowed	44	62	46	27	10	11
Divorced	68	71	17	16	15	13
Never married	48	64	34	26	18	11

Time 1: X^2=25.74, 4 df,	Time 2: X^2=4.87, 4 df, ns
p<.001;

	Women					
	HH, alone		HH, others		Non H, Others	
	Time 1	Time 2	Time 1	Time 2	Time 1	Time 2
Widowed	56	70	36	21	9	8
Divorced	57	69	33	21	10	10
Never married	53	62	25	26	22	12

Time 1: X^2=42.55, 4 df,	Time 2: X^2=7.46, 4 df, ns
p<.001;

	Sex					
Men	53	66	32	23	15	12
Women	55	69	34	22	11	9
Total Sample	55	68	33	22	12	10

Time 1: X^2=4.60, 2 df, ns; Time 2: X^2=2.51, 2 df, ns

to 22 percent at time 2 although this was the second most common living arrangement at both interviews. The proportion of persons who were nonheads of households and living with others changed little from time 1 (12 percent) to time 2 (10 percent). Presumably nonheads of households would include among others the most dependent unmarried aged.

Men and women had similar living arrangements at both time 1 and time 2 (Table 10.3). And, of course, both were more likely to be heads of households and live alone at time 2 than at time 1.

Change in Living Arrangements

Changes shown in Table 10.3 indicate transitions for the group as a whole. By cross-tabulating living arrangements at time 1 by those at time 2, however, it was possible to observe the proportion and direction of change for individuals (Table 10.4).

Living arrangements remained stable for 68 percent of the individuals, whereas 32 percent had changed. Living with others, regardless of whether a person was a head of a household, was a much less stable living arrangement than living alone initially. Almost 90 percent of those who lived alone in their late 50s and early 60s continued to do so ten years later. In contrast, heading a household in which others lived was a stable situation for only 43 percent. Somewhat fewer (38 percent) of those who lived with others but were nonheads of households were in such circumstances a decade later. In a sense, for the majority of individuals living with others and not being a head of household initially did not lead to sustained dependency insofar as this represented the most dependent position.

Thus living alone was the best predictor of doing so as one grew older and the best predictor of stability in living arrangements as well. What directions did the shifts take? Given the categories used, of course, persons who were alone initially could only move to a situation in which they were with others. Persons who shifted from living alone initially most often continued to head a household and had others come into their households (Table 10.4).

In most instances being head of a household would likely connote greater self-sufficiency than living with others as a nonhead. In some situations of extreme dependency, however, individuals may continue to retain their status as household head and employ others to live with them, although for these respondents probably the majority were heads who rented or otherwise shared their quarters.

What happened to those who began the decade as head of a household in which others lived? These persons most often lived alone when they were older. The majority of those who were nonheads of households in their late 50s and early 60s became heads of households by the end of the decade. Thus, even for those in the most dependent situation, the trend was toward independent living. Some of these nonheads of households, as well as heads of households who shifted to living alone, may have been living with their own aged parents.

The transition from being head of a household and living with

Table 10.4
Cross-tabulation of Time 1 by Time 2 Head of Household-Living Arrangements

Time 1 Status	A. Head of Household, Living Alone %	B. Head Household, Living with Others %	C. Nonhead of Household, Living with Others %
A. Head of Household, Living Alone	89 (n=999)	8 (n=92)	3 (n=35)
B. Head of Household, Living with Others	47 (n=319)	43 (n=295)	10 (n=67)
C. Nonhead of Household, Living with Others	33 (n=80)	28 (n=68)	38 (n=92)

others at time 1 to living alone may reflect, in part, that dependent children or grandchildren in the households of some respondents at time 1 had left by the later time. For example, at the beginning of the decade living alone was most popular among both men and women, although the second most frequent living choice among the latter was to live with children or with children and other relatives (24 percent for women compared to 14 percent for men). Men tended to live with other relatives who were not their children (22 percent) and with nonrelatives (9 percent) a little more often than women (16 percent and 4 percent respectively). By the end of the decade, men (4.3 percent) and women (4.6 percent) differed little in their decisions to live with children. Although living with siblings was not common, men chose to live with them (3.5 percent) and nonrelatives (2.4 percent) more frequently than did women (2 percent and 1 percent, respectively). These men never lived with their parents or grandchildren, although a very few women did so (less than 1 percent).

Change in Living Arrangements by Sex

About equal percentages of men and women maintained their living arrangements over the decade with a little over two-thirds continuing in the same living situation at both times (Table 10.3). Women were a little more likely (50 percent) than men (40 percent) to make the most typical shift from living with others as head of a household to living alone. The major difference in the patterns of change of men and women was in the transition from being a nonhead of a household living with others to heading one's own household alone or with others; 38 percent of the men and 22 percent of the women who altered their living arrangements changed in this way. Furthermore, men who became heads of households were more likely to shift from living as nonheads with others to living alone (19 percent compared with 11 percent of women).

Marital Status and Living Arrangements

Marital status was associated with living arrangements at time 1 for both men and women (Table 10.3). Divorced men were much more likely (68 percent) than widowed (44 percent) and never-married men (48 percent) to live alone at time 1. The widowed most often (46 percent) were head of a household and living with others compared with only 17 percent of divorced or 34 percent never married.

This may in part reflect the absence of children with whom the never married might live or that relationships with children may have been severed by the divorced. By time 2, marital status was no longer associated with living arrangements of men; however, percentages of the widowed and never married living alone had increased most (18 and 16 percent respectively). The living arrangements of divorced men changed the least over the decade (Table 10.3).

Marital status made little difference in the tendency for women to live alone at either time 1 or time 2, but it shaped their living arrangements involving others. At time 1, however, widowed and divorced women were a little more likely to be heads of a household living with others than were never-married women; initially, children may have accounted for this difference, but by time 2, never-married women were more often head of a household and living with others than were widowed or divorced women. At the beginning of the decade never-married women were much more likely than other women to be living in a household headed by someone else (22 percent compared with 9 and 10 percent for widowed and divorced, respectively). By the end of the decade, this difference had diminished. Earlier in their lives, never-married women more often may have lived with and cared for an aged parent(s). The never married, especially women, may be caregivers for older, ill, or otherwise dependent relatives. In turn, parents may be a more integral part of the family life of those who never marry.

As observed earlier, in addition to sex and marital status, personal resources such as health, income, and social relationships may prompt decisions for particular living arrangements. In the next sections bivariate relationships between these resources and living arrangements of the unmarried are investigated.

Health and Living Arrangements

Because of the presumed link between health and decisions to live with others, the combined measures used to assess health limitations on mobility and limitations on work and housework in earlier chapters were considered in relation to living arrangements. One-way analyses of variance were employed to investigate relationships between the three types of living arrangements and the combined measures of health status.

An examination of living arrangements in relation to health limitations at time 1 revealed that men who were not heads of households and were living with others reported more health difficulties than men in other arrangements ($F = 3.93$, $p < .05$), although the relationship was not strong. Further tests for differences between groups (i.e., least significant difference test) indicated that heads of households, whether living alone or with others, had comparable health. Female heads of households who lived alone at time 1 were healthier than nonheads, whereas heads of households living with others occupied an intermediate position and did not differ from either of the other groups ($F = 3.90$, $p < .05$).

By the end of the decade, there was a somewhat weaker relationship between health of men and their living arrangements ($F = 2.48$, $p < .10$), although those who were nonheads of households still reported more health difficulties. Health, using the combined items, was not associated with living arrangements among women at time 2 ($F = 1.86$). Percentage differences in health observed between the three types of living arrangements were greater for men than for women. Even so, the most graphic finding was that physical health was not a consistent correlate of living arrangements of the aged.

Use of health services, that is, consulting a physician, hospitalization, and postponement of health care were examined in relation to living arrangements. Among widowed men and women and never-married women health-care behavior was not related to living arrangements. Divorced men and women, however, tended to postpone care more often if they were living with others either as nonhead of a household in the instance of men or if they were heads of households in the instance of women ($\chi^2 = 6.30$, $p < .05$; 4.70, $p < .10$, respectively). Never-married men who lived with others used more health services by receiving care from physicians ($\chi^2 = 4.87$, $p < .10$) and being hospitalized more than their peers who lived alone ($\chi^2 = 6.21$, $p < .05$). As a whole, then, living arrangements were not closely linked to health-care behavior among most of the unmarried and even when living patterns were correlated with use of health care, they were not consistently related across all types of health behavior that were assessed.

Employment and Living Arrangements

Employment status was not associated with living arrangements at either interview for men ($\chi^2 = 1.32$; $.52$). Women who were nonheads of households and living with others were much less likely to be employed (42 percent) than their counterparts who were heads of

households and living alone at time 1 (64 percent; χ^2 = 41.68, p <
.001); however, these differences were no longer evident at time 2
(χ^2 = 3.62, ns).

Income and Living Arrangements

Income was significantly related to living arrangements at both
interviews, although the patterns differed somewhat for men and
women. At both times, female heads of households were more advantaged than nonheads of households whereas those living alone fared
better than their counterparts who headed households and lived with
others (F = 48.57, p < .001; F = 21.85, p < .001).

At time 1, men who headed households regardless of living arrangement were substantially better off than nonheads (F = 5.16, p < .01).
At time 2, however, heads of households who lived with others had
significantly higher incomes than men alone or those who did not
head the households in which they resided (F = 6.01, p < .01). Thus
at the end of the decade women who lived alone continued to be
better off financially, whereas men who headed households but lived
in the company of others were more advantaged.

Childlessness and Living Arrangements

It is clear that for some, having children should expand options for
living arrangements in old age. But what was the effect of children on
the living arrangements of these unmarried men and women? To what
extent were patterns of household composition responsive to the
presence of children or childlessness? And did living arrangements
differ by marital status depending on whether children were available?

Several variations in patterns of living arrangements in relation to
the presence or absence of children were of interest. Living arrangements of divorced men were not affected by having children (χ^2 = .19,
ns). Most of the childless widowers (11 of 13, 85 percent) lived
alone. In contrast, among the widowed fathers, there was more choice
in living arrangements. And one-third of widowed fathers headed
households in which others lived, some of whom would have been
children. Among these unmarried, children likely established themselves in households of their parents more often than parents moved
into the home of children.

Childless widowed women were also more likely to live alone
(81 percent) than the mothers (68 percent, χ^2 = 13.98, p < .001).

Like their male counterparts, a substantial proportion of widowed women with children also ran households in which others resided. Children had a somewhat different effect on the living arrangements of divorced women than for divorced men ($\chi^2 = 6.59$, p $<$ .05). The proportions of divorced women who lived alone differed little by whether they had children (74 percent, childless; 68 percent, parents). But children had an effect on the life-styles of divorced women by influencing whether they lived with others; more than twice as many of the divorced mothers as childless women headed households with others whereas those without children tended to live with others in households that they did not head. Thus the implications of being a parent for living arrangements in later life were somewhat contingent on gender and marital status.

Informal Social Ties and Living Arrangements

Presumably one of the benefits of living in a family or in a setting with others is the availability of potential companions and those with whom to share experiences. Of course, the dominant theme in the literature is that those who live alone will be vulnerable to isolation and will experience deprivation in their social relationships. To assess whether persons living alone were more bereft of interpersonal ties, six measures of informal social relationships were examined in relation to living arrangements in separate one-way analyses of variance for each marital status for men and women. These six measures used in earlier chapters were frequency (never to daily) of face-to-face and telephone contact with neighbors, friends, or relatives (two types of contact by three types of informal associates). Investigation of the six measures of informal association for the three marital statuses resulted in 18 tests each for men and women, or 36 in all.

In general, living arrangements had little effect on the frequency of face-to-face or telephone contact with neighbors, friends, or relatives. Of the 36 analyses of variance, only 11 were significant at the .05 level. Some general patterns, however, were of interest. Frequency of interaction was most often related to the living arrangements of widowed women followed by those of never-married men and women. Living arrangements had no effect on informal social activities of widowed and divorced men, and they had very little influence on the social relationships of divorced women.

Perhaps more important, those who lived alone were *not* more isolated from informal social ties. In instances in which living arrangements were significantly related to informal ties, those who lived alone were most frequently involved with others; a somewhat less common pattern was for heads of households, both those living alone and with others, to have more social interaction than nonheads of households.

Frequency of interaction was most often related to the living arrangements of widowed women followed by those of never-married men and women. Living arrangements had no effect on informal social activities of widowed and divorced men, and they had very little influence on the social relationships of divorced women.

In summary, those living alone were not disproportionately deprived of social ties with others, and in instances, they were advantaged and were able to secure the most contact with neighbors, friends, and relatives. By seeking out others, some of those living alone may have compensated for the isolation their living arrangements might have fostered. The health of those living alone, of course, tended to be at least marginally better than those who were nonheads of households and this may have fostered a somewhat more active social life, especially by the widowed women and the never married of both sexes. It also is possible that the never married and widows living alone always may have affiliated more with others. Heads of households living with others, who usually had fewer social ties than those alone, probably derived some companionship from members of the household and depending on their relationships either may have had less inclination or time to maintain frequent contact with neighbors, friends, or relatives outside the home. Even so, the most important finding was that living alone was not a precursor of social isolation among these unmarried.

Happiness, Satisfaction, and Living Arrangements

In an effort to determine if social psychological well-being was responsive to living arrangements, global happiness and satisfaction with level of activity were considered in relation to living arrangements for the three marital statuses. One-way analyses of variance of happiness and satisfaction with level of activity were calculated for the three marital statuses separately for men and women. Happiness was largely independent of living arrangements for the different marital statuses although widowed men and divorced women who lived alone tended to be happier than their peers with different living arrangements ($F = 3.55$, $p < .05$; $F = 2.32$, $p < .10$, respectively).

Living arrangements were not linked with happiness for the other sex and marital status categories.

Living arrangements were associated with satisfaction with level of activity only among never-married women (F = 3.24, p < .05). Thus it can be concluded that living arrangements had very little influence on two assessments of quality of life for this unmarried sample.

Multivariate Analyses of Living Arrangements

To assess the simultaneous influences of personal resources, discriminant analyses were employed to determine whether those occupying the three types of living arrangements were differentiated by their level of income, health, employment status, race, use of an automobile, presence of children for the formerly married, and happiness. Analyses were conducted separately for men and women and for the different marital statuses (Table 10.5).

Table 10.5
Discriminant Analyses of Living Arrangements at Time 2 for Unmarried Men and Women: Standardized Discriminant Function Coefficients

	Men			Women		
	Widowed	Divorced	Never Married	Widowed	Divorced	Never Married
Income	-.72	.57	.59	-.31	.13	.99
Health	.15	.46	-.90	.01	-.08	-.09
Employment Status	.35	-.80	.11	-.19	-.17	.10
Race	-.42	-.18	---[a]	.13	.75	-.18
Happiness	.41	.34	.07	-.05	.19	.18
Use of Automobile	.59	-.04	.34	.66	-.58	.39
Children	-.14	-.18	---	.40	.68	---
x^2, 14 df	25.60	16.51	22.93	79.76	28.18	24.45
p	.05	ns	.01	.001	.01	.01
Canonical Correlation	.41	.33	.36	.25	.28	.27

[a]Because of the small number of black men among the never married, race was not included.

There was one significant function for each of the sex and marital status groups except for divorced men for whom none of the factors differentiated living arrangements. Income and use of an automobile were the factors that most often distinguished between living arrangements, but they were not always simultaneously important. Income was salient in differentiating among living arrangements of widowed men and never-married men and women. When finances made a difference, the general pattern of income and living arrangements for never-married women and widowed men was such that those who lived alone had higher incomes than nonheads of households. Yet never-married men departed from this pattern since those who lived alone were poorer than heads of households with others in their residence or than those who were nonheads but lived with others. Before a profile of poor, sick, and alone never-married men is drawn, however, it must be noted that health was the strongest predictor of living arrangements of these men. And never-married men who were alone, despite their greater poverty, were most healthy! As observed earlier, never-married men living alone also used health services less frequently. This parallels an earlier finding for this sample in which the physical health of the never married did not seem to be jeopardized by adverse financial circumstances (Keith & Lorenz, 1985). For never-married men this phenomenon appeared to extend to a combined effect of living alone and being poor. In earlier analyses of social ties, health emerged as especially important in the lives of never-married men. Choices of living arrangements of never-married women responded to level of income in a more conventional way because those who resided with others as nonheads of households were also most financially dependent.

Access to private transportation was critical to the living arrangements of much of the sample. Being able to have access to and use of an automobile was the most salient factor for widowed women and to a lesser extent for widowers and divorced women in differentiating whether they were a head of a household, either living alone or with others. Living arrangements of the never married of both sexes were not contingent on access to transportation by private automobile. Except among the never married, however, better health was linked to use of an automobile. Although transportation was a more important direct correlate of living arrangements, for some persons health may have indirectly influenced living arrangements through its association with the ability to use a car.

Even more important than whether they drove and had access to a car, race figured in whether these older divorced women lived alone. Divorced black women were more often in charge of households in which others lived, whereas almost twice as many white divorcees lived alone. This probably reflected a cultural difference in which blacks assume greater responsibility for family members (Brubaker, 1985). In all probability it also revealed joint effects of race and gender, because divorced men tended to select living arrangements that were independent of race, and, furthermore, they were most isolated from significant others with whom they might otherwise have eventually chosen to live or to have live with them. Race was a dimension of importance to living arrangements only among divorced women.

For most, although employment would have affected income that in turn may have made different living arrangements possible, continuing to work was not linked with household patterns. Finally, when other factors were considered simultaneously, happiness did not differentiate among the living arrangements of these unmarried. Thus, happiness was not threatened by a more solitary way of life.

Summary

Which of these findings corroborated or failed to support the literature on factors associated with living arrangements of the aged? Health generally has been found to be a strong predictor of living arrangements although it played a minor part relative to other factors for these unmarried. Health was most important to the never-married men who might have fewer available options to manage physical decline especially less access to assistance typically provided by children. Health may have indirectly affected living arrangements through its precluding or fostering access to private transportation especially among the formerly married. Or maintaining private transportation itself may be an indicator of better functional health.

Common reasoning would suggest that having children could affect the living arrangements of the aged, especially the unmarried. Bachrach (1980) observed that the childless elderly more often lived alone and that living alone resulted in fewer social contacts. We have already seen that living alone did not foster social isolation among these unmarried. The importance of children in determining living arrangements was mitigated by gender, for among these young-old unmarried men and women the childless widowers almost all lived alone, whereas parenthood had no effect on the households of divorced men. Being a mother figured less in whether formerly married women lived alone in later life than in determining their living patterns with others. These findings suggest the importance of considering specific marital statuses as well as the effects of having children in investigations of living arrangements.

PART III: OUTCOMES OF HOMEMAKING, RETIREMENT, AND CONTINUED EMPLOYMENT

In this section, I consider the extent to which these unmarried were vulnerable to financial distress or diminished well-being by virtue of their current employment status (i.e., whether they were employed, retired, or homemakers). In most instances, these three different life-styles in old age reflect decisions made many years earlier. For older women, the outcomes of working versus not working have been studied primarily in terms of which group is most at risk of poor adjustment in retirement. Vulnerability to poorer adjustment is often assessed by differences in social relationships, income, and psychological well-being. In this section, the employed, retired, and homemakers are compared in relation to their finances, satisfaction with activities, and happiness.

Women's changing relationship to the labor force is now well documented, but the transition is nevertheless impressive and carries implications for the unmarried as they age. In the early fifties, 71 percent of women 57 years of age or older were homemakers, 8 percent were retired, and 18 percent were in the labor force. By the late seventies, 40 percent were homemakers, 37 percent were retired, and 20 percent were employed (Riddick, 1985). Increasingly occupational retirement is a role embraced by women even though the proportion who remain employed in later years has been fairly stable.

Considerable speculation about the differential consequences of employment, retirement, and homemaking for the well-being of older women has resulted in comparisons of both objective and subjective indices of well-being for these groups. Much of the speculation about the consequences of retirement for women involves the centrality of homemaking in their lives and the degree to which this involvement will promote adjustment in old age. Recently, O'Rand (1984) observed that the lifetime effects on women of pursuing different roles and different schedules are not yet known.

Evidence from earlier studies provides contradictory conclusions. In a test of the hypothesis that employed women would have higher morale than retired women or homemakers, Jaslow (1976) reported that employed women drawn from a national probability sample had higher morale than retired women when age, health, and income were controlled. When retirees had incomes of $5,000 or more, however, their morale was greater than that of employed women. Homemakers had the lowest morale regardless of controls for age, income, or health. In a study of middle-class Caucasian women, homemakers reported the most positive mental health followed by employed women and retirees (Fox, 1977). More recently Riddick (1985) concluded that employed women enjoyed greater life satisfaction than retirees or homemakers, both of whom tended to report similar levels of well-being. From these studies, it may be concluded that employment status seems to affect well-being of older women although the direction of the effect may be somewhat dependent on income. Furthermore, research based on larger, representative samples provides some evidence that employed older women enjoy somewhat more positive outlooks on life.

The analyses in this section focused on women's labor force involvement and homemaking roles at the end of the decade. By the close of the decade, 720 women described themselves as homemakers, 605 retired, and 208 employed. Fifty-seven percent (n = 954) of the unmarried women had been employed at the beginning of the decade whereas 12 percent (n = 208) were still in the labor force at completion of the study.

Since income over the life cycle is related to work history and is reflected in resources available and level of living in later years, the employed, retired, and homemakers were compared on five indices including financial dimensions; these were satisfaction with level of living, financial hardship (ability to get along on present income), actual income, appraisals of global happiness, and satisfaction with level of activity.

RESULTS

Women who remained employed later in life fared better on all indices than homemakers, and they were generally better off than the retired on four of the five measures (Table 10.6). In turn, the retired tended to view their situations more positively than homemakers did on four of the indices.

Employed women were more satisfied with their level of living, were better able to get along with less financial hardship, and enjoyed

Table 10.6
Mean Values, F and T Values for Finances and Well-Being
by Employment Status of Women

Finances and Well-being	Mean Values Women			F
	Employed (1)	Retired (2)	Homemakers (3)	
	X	X	X	
Satisfaction with level of living	2.90	2.73	2.63	13.63 (<.001) 3 < 1,2 2 < 1
Financial adequacy	2.72	2.45	2.21	29.63 (<.001) 3 < 1,2 2 < 1
Income	10.30	8.76	7.31	47.48 (<.001) 3 < 1,2 2 < 1
Happiness	2.24	2.15	2.04	9.26 (<.001) 3 < 1,2
Satisfaction with level of activity	3.01	2.81	2.77	11.44 (<.001) 1 < 2,3

larger incomes than both homemakers and retired women. Although employed women were happier than homemakers, they did not express greater happiness than the retired. At the same time, the retired were more satisifed with their level of living, had less financial hardship, were happier, and had higher incomes than homemakers.

Clearly, labor force involvement, both current and former, differentiated the lives of these unmarried women in old age. Although women who continued to work were in better financial circumstances and were more satisfied with their level of activity than the retired, the somewhat less advantageous economic situations of the latter did not preclude them from achieving happiness equal to that of the employed. Homemakers' lives were considerably more fraught with financial distress and unhappiness.

PART IV: CHILDLESSNESS

In this section, the consequences of childlessness for formerly married men and women are considered. Childlessness is included in a chapter on vulnerability because in old age not being a parent is seen as leaving individuals at greater risk of loneliness and bereft of a potentially major support system. For those without spouses, childlessness means that yet another possible social tie is not available.

Norms of filial responsibility and reciprocal exchanges between parents and children are evident throughout the life cycle. Parents and adult children maintain interpersonal relationships and exchange advice, emergency assistance, and goods and services across the years. Adults usually endorse notions of filial responsibility although much aid that flows between children and their aged parents is mutual with both helping the other but with diverse kinds of assistance. It has been observed that middle-aged children who care for an aged parent may do so with the hope that they will be a model for their own children who in time will not abandon them when they are old. Certainly reasons given for having children include their potential contribution of caring and assistance in their parents' old age. In fact, some research has shown that as persons age they tend to expect greater aid and support from children (Seelbach, 1978), although older persons seem to prefer affective and social relationships more than instrumental or economic support (Seelbach & Sauer, 1977). This is consonant with the finding that the aged would rather engage professionals to provide instrumental care than to depend on family members (Lee, 1985). When aid is given, however, children are in the forefront in providing personal care and assistance. That children clearly make a tangible or intangible contribution to the lives of many older persons raises the question of how the childless manage in later life and whether they fare less well than their age peers who are parents.

One thesis in the literature implies that the childless will be disadvantaged and encounter difficulties. As noted in Chapter 1, this perspective posits that like singleness, childlessness is an atypical family pattern. As a deviant status, childlessness may require strategies for management not required of parents. This view includes the thought that "having children is good insurance against loneliness and isolation in old age" (Glenn & McLanahan, 1981:410) and that not having them leads to deprivation.

A contrasting perspective speculates that the childless develop strategies for coping in the absence of children. Never expecting that they will have a relationship with an adult child in their old age, they develop competencies and relationships independent of children. In their accommodation to the absence of children then, the childless may capitalize on the opportunities to establish and maintain friendships, become involved in community associations, and in nonwork activities that the presence of children might curtail (Glenn & McLanahan, 1981). Bachrach (1980) found that when the childless enjoyed good health, they were more likely to have had recent contact with friends and neighbors than were parents. Moreover, the high level of nonkin contact diminished isolation and by and large offset the absence of interaction with children. Although she found that isolation occurred more often for the childless in poor health and those with working-class backgrounds, further possible links between childlessness and psychological outcomes were not examined. What does seem to be the contribution of children to the psychological well-being of older parents?

In spite of any potential benefits derived from the mutual fulfillment of filial responsibilities in later life, there is evidence of some negative effects of children on the psychological well-being of parents earlier in the life cycle (Glenn & McLanahan, 1982). It has been suggested, however, that the benefits of children may be more obvious in middle and later life when interaction may be enjoyable and accompanied with less parental responsibility. Yet, the investigation by Glenn and McLanahan (1981:409) of persons age 50 or over provided "little evidence that important psychological rewards are derived from the later stages of parenthood." Furthermore, the effects of children on global happiness were negligible or negative.

There is some suggestion that affiliation with children may have somewhat different outcomes for older men and women. O'Rand (1984), for example, observed that children have a positive effect on women's adjustment whereas they do not influence men's lives in the same way. O'Rand (1984:136) concluded that "Paradoxically, women's family roles negatively influence their work careers and earning capacities in earlier phases of their lives, but have positive returns to women in old age when noneconomic resources provided by children enhance women's lives."

Thus the consequences of not having children in old age are not entirely clear. On the one hand for a minority of the aged who need extensive assistance, children provide a considerable proportion of help that is received. Less is known about how the childless, unmarried manage in old age when needs for assistance may be at their greatest. In this research, data were not available on all of the specific kinds of help parents may have given to or received from children, but it was possible to obtain a comparative glimpse of how other resources may have varied for parents and the childless over the decade. Keeping in mind that the divorced and widowed may reach old age with different kinds of relationships with their adult children, comparisons were made between parents and childless men and women who were widowed and divorced.

RESULTS

Socioeconomic Resources of Parents and the Childless

Income at the beginning and end of the decade as well as education were considered in relation to the presence and absence of children. T-tests were used to assess differences in resources between parents and the childless. To determine whether the effects of childlessness might vary by marital status and gender analyses were conducted separately for the widowed and divorced and for men and women.

Educational levels of widowed and divorced men were independent of whether they had children ($t = 1.09$; .10, respectively). Income both earlier in their lives ($t = 1.30$, .11) and later at time 2 was similar regardless of whether they were parents ($t = 1.36$, .70).

Having children, however, was more strongly correlated with the resources of women because childless widowed and divorced women had higher levels of education than their peers who were mothers ($t = 3.07$, $p < .01$; $t = 2.17$, $p < .05$, respectively). Earlier in their lives, but not later, childless widowed women had higher incomes ($t = 3.04$, $p < .01$; $t = 1.53$, times 1 and 2, respectively). The presence of children was not associated with the incomes of divorced women at either the beginning or the end of the decade ($t = .05$; $t = 1.18$, times 1 and 2, respectively). It should also be noted that children did not depress participation of women in the labor force at the time of either interview although they may have constrained employment earlier when their mothers were substantially younger.

Health of Parents and the Childless

Self-rated health was studied in relation to the presence or absence of children. The health of widowed and divorced men was not associated with the presence of children at either time 1 ($t = .16$, .74, widowed, divorced, respectively) or time 2 ($t = .04$, 1.63). Widowed and divorced women with children had somewhat better health than their childless counterparts earlier in their lives ($t = 2.41$, $p < .05$; 1.88, $p < .10$) but not when they were older ($t = .14$; 1.79, widowed and divorced, respectively).

Affiliation and Well-Being of Parents and the Childless

For the most part, the childless were not more active in formal organizations at the end of the decade ($t = .68$, .13, widowed men and women; $t = .39$, divorced men). Childless divorced women, however, participated somewhat more in formal organizations than their counterparts who were parents ($t = 2.14$, $p < .05$).

The relationship between parental status and informal ties varied most by gender. Childless divorced and widowed women saw their siblings more often ($t = 2.23$, $p < .05$; 1.96, $p < .05$) and tended to have more frequent contact with friends ($t = 1.91$, $p < .06$; 2.85, $p < .01$) than their peers who were mothers. Like the widowed men ($t = 1.95$, $p < .05$) and women ($t = 5.60$, $p < .001$), divorcees without children had less interaction with relatives (2.57, $p < .01$).

Divorced and widowed men maintained social ties with siblings ($t = .36$; 1.05) and friends ($t = .26$; .50) independently of whether they had children. Perhaps further indicating how little their children impinged on the lives of these divorced men their contact with relatives was not linked to whether they were parents ($t = .94$).

Finally, to respond, in part, to the view that the childless will be bereft and unhappier than parents in their old age, I compared happiness and satisfaction with level of activity of the formerly married who were parents and those who were childless. Both earlier in their lives and at the end of the decade the formerly married childless were just as happy and as satisfied with the amount of activity as were parents.

Although children may have had a depressing effect on the earlier educational attainments of both widowed and divorced women and the income of widowed women, in old age children had most influence on the nature of the social lives of the formerly married women. The social relationships of men were conducted by and large independently of having children. Formerly married women without children available may have compensated by seeking our further informal contacts, or perhaps opportunities to be with children diminished the association of mothers with friends or others.

Even though on most measures used here these unmarried aged with children were not differentiated from their childless peers, it is known that the reciprocity and exchanges of goods, services, and mutual support referred to earlier in this section characterize the relationships of many older parents and their adult children. It was possible to obtain a limited view of these exchanges through the monetary contributions parents and children made to one another over time.

Across the decade these unmarried aged decreased the support they gave to children. This probably reflected the presence of young adult children still living in the home at the time of the earliest interview. When they were in their early 60s, 11 percent of the unmarried women and 22 percent of the men assisted their children with either partial or complete support. Ten years later, the proportion who provided support to their children had declined markedly with only 5 percent of the men and 4 percent of the women contributing to the finances of their children.

As the literature suggests, however, some parents also received help from their children. At both the beginning and end of the decade substantially more women (20 percent) than men (6 percent) received at least some support from their children. Ten years later more women still obtained help, although it had declined somewhat with 16 percent having some support from children compared with 7 percent of the men. In summary, patterns of monetary exchange over time indicated that support to children declined over the decade whereas assistance given to parents was more consistent, although that provided to women diminished somewhat. Thus any decline in income with retirement was not offset by an increased flow of support from children to parents. Finally, these formerly married women were recipients of support two to three times more often than their male peers. In any event, a minority of both men and women consistently were beneficiaries of help from children that would have been unavailable to their childless peers. Even so, monetary assistance from children did not elevate the incomes of parents above those of the childless.

Further analyses considered the relationship between giving and receiving aid and well-being as assessed by happiness. It has been observed that receiving assistance from significant others may erode the satisfaction and morale of older persons (Lee, 1985). Neither giving nor receiving assistance from children was linked to happiness or satisfaction with level of living of these unmarried. Any benefit accruing to these aged or any feelings of being unable to reciprocate were not reflected in either increased or diminished happiness. Consequently, such exchanges seemed to be benign for these older unmarried parents.

SUMMARY AND CONCLUSIONS

This chapter has demonstrated that only under certain conditions did phenomena often identified as fostering vulnerability in the elderly put these unmarried at greater risk of incurring diminished well-being. By considering both social isolation and living alone, this chapter has addressed the common reasoning that older persons, perhaps especially the unmarried, are alone, and that being alone has undesirable consequences for the quality of life.

Social isolation was not synonymous with dissatisfaction, feelings of deprivation, or disadvantaged circumstances. Rather, the congruence between preferences and the relationships that the aged were able to maintain tended to be crucial in differentiating those most vulnerable to diminished resources and unhappiness. Likewise, when the unmarried lived alone, their contacts with others either thrived or certainly were not diminished. Furthermore, neither happiness nor satisfaction with the level of their activities were thwarted by living alone, perhaps supporting the view that household composition is not a good indicator of the quality of social interaction (Fischer & Phillips, 1982). Although findings such as these are somewhat counterintuitive, other research has failed to provide substantial support for the popular thinking that being alone is equivalent to loneliness; indeed, older persons are not especially lonely (Fischer & Phillips, 1982), even though many do not live with others.

As noted earlier, for the unmarried childlessness likely reduces potential sources of support, opportunities for companionship, and possibly diminishes residential options. Having children made little difference in the resources, financial or social, or in the happiness of these fathers and mothers. Although a minority of these older, unmarried parents received some financial assistance from children, it did not affect their feelings of financial hardship or their evaluations of their lives as reflected in happiness and satisfaction. Of course, some of the parents lived with their children, an option that the childless would not have. More often than not, however, in fact more than twice as frequently, parents were heads of households in which others lived rather than residing in the homes of their children. Thus few parents were living as nonheads of households in their children's residences. In summary, granted that some of the measures, especially the social psychological indices, were limited, the findings corroborated other literature suggesting that childlessness, for the most part, tends to be benign.

Having been employed earlier in their lives continued to have positive consequences for these unmarried women as much as a decade later. But remaining employed into their late 60s and early 70s was beneficial for these unmarried women relative to the quality of life experienced by their retired and homemaker peers. Although employment may have occurred much earlier in their lives, advantages continued to accrue to the retired over those enjoyed by homemakers. Of the three groups, the homemakers were the most vulnerable to financial hardship, dissatisfaction with their level of living and activity, and greater unhappiness. In fairness, however, it should be remembered that many of the measures used were related to aspects of finances in which the employed and retired were more advantaged. Even so, one conclusion from these analyses is that selected factors sometimes believed to increase the risk of a diminished quality of life in old age perhaps may affect only a minority and then only under certain conditions.

Concluding Thoughts

11

An intent of this chapter is to summarize and comment on some of the implications of outcomes in various spheres of life among the unmarried. Figuring more prominently in some areas of life than others, marital status generally had stronger effects for women than for men. These women's lives especially were shaped by the decision never to marry or perhaps by characteristics that predisposed them to remain single initially. In contrast, outcomes for men were more often differentiated from those of others by divorce.

HEALTH

Health was the linchpin that was reflected in both the tangible and nonmaterial products of their lives. The health of these unmarried had deteriorated over the decade but even then the majority did not have a health problem that limited how well they got around or one that interfered with work or housework. Indeed, a majority continued to describe their health as the "same as or better than" that of their age peers.

To the degree that marital status was linked with health among the unmarried, there were sharper differences found among women. Across a number of indices, never-married women had fewer health limitations and difficulties whereas divorced men were impaired most often or experienced increases in physical disability over the decade more than any other group. In general, widowers and never-married men were more alike in the health they enjoyed while widows and divorced women had more comparable assessments of their health. Perhaps some of the benefits of marriage believed to be greater for men than for women continued to favor widowers and were reflected in their health later. Possible reasons that the health of never-married men was less differentiated from that of other men in contrast to more marked differences found between never-married and formerly married women, in part, may be attributed to variations in conditions that selected them into singleness initially or perhaps their lesser ability to manage their marital status as well as women did.

Postponement of needed treatment is illustrative of one type of health care behavior. Marital status was especially linked to reasons for postponement of needed health care. Obtaining care readily and without delay may decrease the probability of developing or at least mitigate the effects of chronic diseases and disability in later life. Finances were important factors in the failure to seek care. The decisions of the never married to obtain care were least influenced by economic circumstances and were more often dominated by emotional reasons. Both economic and emotional dimensions of health care decisions should be amenable to intervention. The persistence of these barriers to health care over time suggests that intervention should be introduced early in the life cycle.

Finally, whereas financial hardship and economic strain were important in seeking or postponing health care, they had a less direct effect on assessments of physical health. Furthermore, there was no evidence that being worried and dispirited about economic circumstances eroded health over time (Keith & Lorenz, 1985). A future model should include the effects of economic affairs on postponement of health care and in turn its effect on multiple measures of physical and mental health. Understanding the possible effects of marital status in relation to health care behavior must take into account that the factors apparently motivating these never married, both men and women, were somewhat differentiated from those that prompted health care activities of the formerly married.

Two pieces of data allude to the suggestion, although perhaps subtly, that the never married may have exhibited divergent health behaviors and maybe even arrived at assessments of their health under dissimilar circumstances than the formerly married. One involved the tendency to maintain good health despite financial circumstances that might have fostered illness in others (Keith & Lorenz, 1985). The other referred to the importance of emotional reasons for not seeking health care reported by both never-married men and women.

Although speculative, other analyses of these data suggested that assessments of health by some of the never-married men and women may involve construction of positive evaluations despite hardship and distress over financial circumstances (Keith & Lorenz, 1985). Some never-married men and women with greater financial strain and hardship over the decade actually enjoyed better health at the end of the ten-year period. The never married may reflect a kind of hardiness resulting from the sustained development of independence over their life course. Perhaps the emotional reasons they listed as reasons for postponing or not obtaining care may have enabled them to persist and even thrive in the face of other difficulties. Health may be especially important to the never married who are likely to confront old age with fewer sources of support or at least those that may languish in the face of diminished physical mobility. Health is most critical to a successful single life-style. Bachrach (1980) observed that health differentiated singles who maintained richer lives from those who were lonely.

AFFILIATION WITH SIGNIFICANT OTHERS

The specter of reaching old age and being alone is vividly presented in popular literature and until recently, although to a lesser extent, in scientific writing. Furthermore, a hidden assumption, although one that is infrequently tested, is that isolation increases precipitously with aging. What changes occurred in the social lives of these older unmarried men and women over time? How did marital status and gender figure in the patterns and changes in their social ties?

Most of these unmarried aged were not isolated from contact with friends and family. Social isolation was not synonymous with dissatisfaction, feelings of deprivation, disadvantaged circumstances or even living alone. Rather, incongruence between their preferences and their actual social relationships was more often linked to diminished resources and unhappiness. Moreover, neither happiness nor satisfaction with their level of activities were thwarted by living alone. Indeed, for some there may have been slight advantages in happiness accruing to those who lived alone.

Generally, childlessness was benign in its impact on the lives of these older formerly married men and women. Its effects were somewhat greater for divorced and widowed women, who when childless, were integrated into networks of siblings and friends more often than were mothers. This may have represented compensation for the absence of children with whom to affiliate. For the most part, the social lives of widowed and divorced men were less affected by having children.

Marital status differentiated some of the opportunities for social relationships. From the standpoint of information for practice, perhaps one of the most graphic findings was that almost one-half of the divorced men either had no children or were estranged from them. This likely reflected the effects of both gender and marital status since formerly married men had less frequent contact with children than did women, and divorce may be a more alienating experience from the family for men than for women. Should these men require care in the face of severe illness, siblings, friends, or formal organizations will be needed. Other research has shown that the unmarried, and men in particular, draw more heavily on extra family sources of assistance.

How did the social relationships of these unmarried change over time? The unmarried were not increasingly isolated from their children because most maintained stable relationships with them over the decade. For the majority of those who incurred change, it signaled more contact with children, except for divorced men.

Contrasting with the increases in affiliation with children, transitions in relationships with siblings and friends were usually harbingers of declines in contact. This finding is critical since friends more often than family are demonstrated to have positive effects on well-being in old age (Lee, 1985). Furthermore, whereas there are a finite number of available family members, potential new friends might be more abundant. Yet, compared to ties with family, friendships were less stable and most often declined when they did change. Never-married men and women were most accomplished at augmenting their friendships in later life.

Plans for intervention to enhance informal interaction of the unmarried aged might be guided somewhat by knowledge of the characteristics that fostered contact. In general, prior levels of affiliation were most salient in determining participation later in life. Social lives of women were shaped more by socioeconomic factors than were the relationships that men maintained with others although the interaction of divorced and never-married men was more responsive to socioeconomic status than that of widowed men. Women's friendships seemed to be especially vulnerable to financial circumstances. Never-married women were favored by more friendship ties, but these and their relationships with siblings were tempered by dimensions of social class so that poorer women were less advantaged. If financial resources are eroded in later life, perhaps by poor health and medical expenditures, social ties of women, particularly those of the never married, likely would be curtailed the most.

Because social ties external to the household are of undoubted importance to the unmarried, questions often are asked about who has the most contact with family and friends—men or women? Recent literature, of course, has defined women as keepers of the kin and their tendency to form close relationships with friends as well has been documented. Do these differences persist outside of marriage and into later life? If there are gender differences between spouses in maintaining family ties, are they also apparent among the unmarried?

Among these unmarried, there were no consistent patterns of gender differences in contact with siblings at the beginning and end of a decade within the marital statuses. Of the six tests (3 marital statuses by involvement with siblings at time 1 and time 2), there were gender differences in only two instances, both of which favored greater involvement by women. It must be concluded that gender was not a primary factor in differentiating contact with brothers and sisters by these unmarried men and women.

Compared with their association with siblings, ties with friends were more responsive to gender. Although I could not assess the relative closeness that men and women felt toward their friends, the amount of contact of these unmarrieds with their friends generally conformed to findings in the literature. That is, women maintained more contact with their friends than did men especially when they were older. At the end of the decade this gender difference was evident regardless of marital status. A similar pattern was observed for the contact of the formerly married with their children. Thus, association with siblings seemed to be the one area in which women did not maintain the most involvement with others. These findings then suggest that perhaps the generalization of Adams (1968) about women's greater ties with kin compared with those of men should be amended to take into account marital status and type of kin.

LEISURE ACTIVITIES OF THE UNMARRIED

Involvement in in-home and out-of-home leisure activities over a four-year period was quite stable for this group of unmarried persons as a whole. Gender differences in leisure pursuits were marked and should be attended to by those interested in planning programs for older men and women. It could not be concluded, however, that most leisure activities of men and women were quite distinct; rather, there was overlapping involvement in the majority of pursuits. Marital status was less important than gender in determining how the unmarried spent their time. Again some of the distinctiveness of the lives of never-married women was manifested in their greater participation in activities outside the home. These women who had never had the competing demands of spouses and children, although a minority may have cared for parents, developed more outreach activities into the community through formal participation than their formerly married peers.

As they develop programs for the aged, planners may want to consider some of the distinctions between levels of involvement of the unmarried in rural and urban areas. Place of residence figured in the tendency to participate in particular types of activities as well. Generally urban women were most integrated into their communities through social participation and perhaps capitalized on the greater diversity of the environment in ways that their unmarried male counterparts did not. These unmarried rural men and women were more disadvantaged in income and education compared to those living in cities. Furthermore, formal and informal involvement was constrained by low income. Rural men were least involved across most activities, and their participation especially was limited by poor health and income. To the extent possible planners will want to ensure there are opportunities for participation that are independent of income.

Those who advocate focusing on leisure activities as a part of preretirement programming suggest that such pursuits will contribute to psychological well-being. What conclusions can be drawn about the specific activities engaged in that brought the most happiness and satisfaction to these unmarried people? And were these activities among the most frequently undertaken? First, none of the activities consistently fostered happiness and satisfaction across all groups, although hobbies, more than any other in-home activities, were often a source of well-being.

Participation in senior centers, which in itself was not a source of well-being, could be used to teach some of the skills that result in leisure activities that in turn contribute to happiness and satisfaction. Efforts should be made to increase participation especially by men. The importance of volunteer work in fostering well-being among these unmarried suggests that efforts should be made to involve them in a

greater way in these activities. As well as providing men with opportunities to use their existing skills, volunteering also will benefit communities. Practitioners will want to make an effort to ensure that
volunteer opportunities are available in rural areas and extend special
encouragement for involvement by men for whom the activity was
especially satisfying.

Place of residence made a difference in the activities of the unmarried although gender continued to exert a strong influence irrespective
of size of community. Those who plan programs for older adults,
regardless of marital status, should make decisions taking into account
both gender and size of place.

FINANCES

Investigation of the financial situation of these unmarried women
echoed findings for other areas of life by indicating the greater difficulties of the widowed and divorced relative to the never married.
For example, formerly married women fared less well than the never
married in both amount of income and the financial hardship they
experienced. Divorce, but not widowhood, seemed to have a negative
effect on the financial circumstances of men especially by the end of
the decade. Race also was especially important in determining the
extent of financial hardship of divorced men. For these men there
was the combined difficulty of being a member of a minority group
and of being divorced that contributed to difficulties in managing
their economic circumstances that were not experienced by widowed
men, either black or white. Both objectively, as reflected in lower
income, and subjectively as in observations of hardship and dissatisfaction with their conditions, divorced men were least advantaged
and the most troubled of all men.

Actual income seemed to impact satisfaction with level of living
through its effect on feelings of hardship. Race and income interacted in such a way that black formerly married men and women
with higher incomes were less satisfied with their level of living than
white men and women with comparable incomes. A parallel finding
was observed for financial hardship among never-married women
because high-income black women viewed their financial situation as
more precarious and difficult than white women with substantially
lower incomes and who were objectively much worse off. There may
have been more demands on the incomes of blacks than whites for
intergenerational support and other contributions to extended family

members. These demands may have eroded their satisfaction and among never-married minority women may have fostered financial hardship. Perhaps because they were seen as having fewer claims on their income, never-married black women with high salaries or wages may have been especially vulnerable to requests for assistance and expectations that they meet the needs of family members. Another possible explanation for the seeming discrepancy between amount of income and difficulty making ends meet identified by the subgroup of unmarried blacks may be that their expectations for their own prosperity may have exceeded what they were able to attain. The inconsistency between what some blacks achieved and the difficulty with which they managed their financial circumstances may have prompted the substantially higher rates of employment of divorced men and women later in their lives compared with some of the other unmarried persons.

The early anticipation of financial problems in retirement reached across the years in the lives of these unmarried. At the beginning of the decade, black women and especially the divorced were plagued by the expectation of financial difficulties in retirement. And their fears and those of others were not groundless, for both men and women who expected problems ten years earlier were more dissatisfied with their level of living and experienced considerably greater financial hardship at the close of the decade.

Moreover, those who address the needs of divorced women will want to realize not only the substantial contribution of paid employment to the income of these women but also the benefit of work late in their lives in reducing feelings of financial hardship. Even in their late 60s and early 70s employment sustained divorced women in ways that it did not other unmarried men or women.

The consequences of being unmarried in old age for the financial domain of life were that the strains of divorce and widowhood for women and divorce for men had an enduring negative influence over the decade, if not an increasing impact over time for the latter group. Although Zick and Smith (1986) found that widowers as well as widows experienced a loss in income, the hardship of these widowers relative to that of the divorced was somewhat less.

WORK AND RETIREMENT

What did research reveal about the work and retirement orientations of these unmarried men and women? Did women have more difficulty accepting retirement? Were never-married women more reluctant to retire than their formerly married peers? Earlier research presumed that women would find retirement easier than men would whereas some recent investigations have indicated women are more negative toward retirement (Gee & Kimball, 1987).

Whether women's assessments of work and retirement differed from those of men was contingent on marital status. Formerly married men held more positive evaluations of both work and retirement than did widowed and divorced women across the decade. By the end of the decade never-married men and women had similar views of work and women tended to be slightly more favorable toward retirement. Thus the argument that women will be less positively predisposed to retirement than men received support only among the formerly married. These women also had more limited economic resources than the never married and may have been responding to the negative aspects of even further diminished finances in retirement. Never-married women embraced retirement, and, thus, did not confirm the thinking that those who have never married and have had sustained careers may have greater difficulties adjusting to retirement.

Never-married women were employed in higher status occupations than the formerly married. It has been observed in other research that attitudes toward retirement held by professional women are predicted more by employment factors whereas attitudes of nonprofessional women are more often determined by financial circumstances (Gee & Kimball, 1987).

Positive attitudes toward retirement were especially important to the happiness of women. Indeed, for many in the sample, feelings about retirement were more closely linked with later happiness than were earlier assessments of happiness. Yet, especially for divorced women, the prospect of happiness in their retirement years was jeopardized by earlier expectations of financial hardships.

HOUSEHOLD INVOLVEMENT

In their involvement in the household, the lives of unmarried men and women remained quite divergent. Men clearly made more alternative arrangements for managing some of the "feminine" activities that women were likely to do for themselves. These people counted on children, friends, and hired persons when they needed help with less assistance from grandchildren, siblings, and more distant relatives. For most activities women relied more on hired services than did men, who received a little more help on most household tasks from children and friends. As might be expected, having children who lived in closer proximity was associated with receiving more help.

Not surprisingly, better health prompted greater involvement in the household by both men and women. And in turn, household involvement was modestly related to life satisfaction. Thus performance of primarily "feminine" tasks was not disadvantageous to men nor did it detract from the well-being of women.

HAPPINESS OF THE UNMARRIED

A remaining question is how gender and marital status were linked with happiness among these unmarried men and women and which factors seemed to contribute to positive outlooks on life. First, results of bivariate analyses of marital status, gender, and happiness are considered. Second, to place multivariate models of happiness in context, theories and frameworks used by gerontologists to explain differences in assessments of later life are reviewed briefly. Finally, outcomes of multivariate analyses described in earlier chapters and a concluding analysis of happiness are discussed.

These unmarried men more often than women said they were not too happy (25 percent vs. 18 percent). Yet this did not mean that happiness of men had eroded over time, because actually slightly fewer were very unhappy at the end of the decade than earlier (28 percent, time 1 compared to 25 percent, time 2). Somewhat more women (25 percent) reported that they were pretty happy than did men (21 percent). Even so, about one-fifth to one-quarter of these men and women were in the extreme categories of happiness, reporting being either unhappy or very happy.

At time 1, marital status was not associated with the happiness of men ($F = 1.71$, ns). By the end of the decade, however, never-married men tended to report greater happiness than the divorced ($F = 2.80$, $p < .06$) with ratings of widowed men falling in between. Never-married women enjoyed greater happiness than widowed and divorced women at both interviews ($F = 16.24$, $p < .001$; 7.24, $p < .001$). Gee & Kimball (1987) also remarked on the higher satisfaction of never-married women compared to their formerly married peers. In fact, never-married women reported substantially greater happiness than any of these other unmarried persons. We need to ask what factors contributed to their more appreciative views of their lives. That is, which, if any, of the dimensions studied here seemed to account for their more positive reviews of their circumstances?

PERSPECTIVES ON OUTLOOKS ON LIFE IN OLD AGE

Change in Marital Status

Much research in social gerontology has focused on the prediction of life satisfaction and positive adjustment among the aged. And there has been considerable popular and scientific speculation about the origins and correlates of happiness and psychological well-being in later life. Change in marital status has been a critical variable in some of these investigations with primary comparisons made between the widowed and the married. Various theoretical frameworks offer contrasting views of the factors that prompt satisfaction in later life. Role, activity, and stress theories suggest that widowhood will decrease life satisfaction. Network exchange theories posit that transitions such as widowhood and divorce alter opportunities for achieving gratifying relationships in old age.

Role theory indicates that widowhood represents a loss typical and expected in old age. Yet losing a role and a primary relationship even though it may be anticipated disrupts established patterns of behavior, modifies individual self identity, even age identification, and results in differential treatment received from other persons.

Activity theory predicts that total activity is lessened with role loss and, in turn, opportunities for others to validate specific role identities and self-concept are reduced. An outcome of this process is that positive self-concept may be eroded and appreciative feelings about life as a whole decline.

One stress model posits that unpleasant and discomforting role losses are stressors that directly reduce subjective well-being (Elwell & Maltbie-Crannell, 1981). These same losses may contract resources such as income, health, and social support, and both directly and indirectly, erode well-being. Therefore, these three frameworks postulate that declines in morale, happiness, and other outlooks on life occur following reductions in roles and resources.

Network exchange theory assumes that transitions in status like divorce or widowhood alter opportunities, costs, rewards, and benefits that eventually affect lifestyle and contentment (Dowd, 1980). According to this approach, despair, despondency, and unhappiness are not expected conditions of old age; rather, resources and the competency in negotiating rewarding exchanges will shape the circumstances of later life. For the most part, these frameworks—role, activity, stress, and exchange theories—each postulate that divorce and widowhood may foster discontentment in old age although the mechanism by which subjective well-being is altered differs.

Well-Being, Role Loss, and Resources

Although widowed and divorced persons usually report lower life satisfaction and happiness than married individuals, role, activity, stress, and exchange approaches propose a number of factors that may mediate between the effects of marital status and subjective appraisals of life. Differences in the amount of pleasure persons derive from life, however, may be more contingent on socioeconomic factors and health than marital status alone (Larson, 1978). Of course, as noted earlier, finances and health also are linked with marital status.

A core notion in an exchange network perspective is that social networks impact individual attitudes and values as well as interpersonal ties. As observed in Chapter 9, both community and network attributes shape opportunities for and constraints on interaction with others. Sibling, child, and friend interaction may form the basis for considerable social support and help to the unmarried in old age (Chapters 7 and 8). Both amount and intimacy of informal interaction are believed to facilitate adjustment. For example, Shanas (1980) has described the family as a "safe harbor" and a "basis for security" in old age. She supports her claim with evidence that family, especially children, reside close by, visit regularly, assist with chores, and maintain emotional bonds with aging adults. Activity and stress theories both endorse family interaction as a form of social support and posit that informal interaction with relatives will enhance life satisfaction (Elwell & Maltbie-Crannell, 1981; Mouser et al., 1985). As was observed in Chapter 8, however, there are reasons why child and sibling interaction may be less preferable to friend contact as a source of support (Lee, 1985). Or an exchange perspective would suggest caution in expecting the highest reward from child interaction.

When changes occur, such as retirement, widowhood, and divorce, other resources, like energy, health, and income, may diminish as well and decrease opportunities to renegotiate rewarding exchanges. Family interaction, for example, may be shaped by dwindling parental resources with children assuming more responsibility for care and decision making. The new interaction patterns may highlight a power shift or even dependency on the part of the parent. Exchanges with children may be less enjoyable and rewarding with the outcome that extensive child contact depresses morale and satisfaction of both children and their parents.

An assumption of network exchange theory is that persons try to maintain satisfying exchanges and insofar as possible avoid unpleasant ones. Age peers, in contrast to children, may provide more opportunities for rewarding and balanced exchanges because they share comparable interests, life experiences, and resources (Dowd, 1980). One of the more consistent research findings is the importance of voluntary interaction with friends to enjoyment and contentment with life of older persons (Mouser et al., 1985).

Some of the factors that motivate and provide rewards from interaction with friends may be those that also foster involvement in formal organizations. Since organizational affiliations are not compulsory, older persons likely retain those that provide rewards. The positive outcomes may include opportunities to learn new things, involvement in interesting activities, enhancement of self esteem, and acquisition of social support. Reaping such rewards may account for the considerable continuity in ties with formal organizations among these unmarried as observed in Chapter 8. Much research has confirmed the contribution of participation in formal organizations to life satisfaction (see Mouser et al., 1985, for a review).

Although retirement is a role loss, there is some evidence that negative effects may be attributable less to withdrawal from work itself than to health problems, diminished income, early and involuntary retirement, lack of preparation, and perhaps poorer adjustment prior to ceasing employment. Opportunities for happiness are not dissimilar for retirees and employees when some of these factors are taken into account (Beck, 1982).

Following from exchange theory, health and financial status are indices of opportunities to negotiate rewarding exchanges that may reduce stress and facilitate well-being (Mouser et al., 1985) and are usually among the best indicators of subjective assessments of adjustment. As noted in earlier chapters, income may indirectly affect estimates of well-being by influencing perceptions of hardship and financial adequacy. Financial circumstances may indirectly influence well-being by providing options for the use of leisure time and interpersonal involvement. As shown in Chapter 9, formal and informal ties of these unmarried, regardless of rural or urban place of residence, were constrained somewhat by income.

Education is also an aspect of socioeconomic resources that may directly or indirectly affect subjective well-being because it is reflected in social skills, problem solving, choices of leisure activities, and development of friendships and social support. As indicated in Chapter 9, education particularly influenced the leisure involvement and happiness of rural unmarried women.

CONCLUSIONS FROM MULTIVARIATE MODELS

Thus, a number of personal resources may contribute to happiness in old age and may mediate between marital status and well-being. Several analyses provided information on the happiness of these unmarried: (a) the importance of attitudes toward retirement in fostering happiness (Chapter 5); (b) comparisons of correlates of well-being of rural and urban residents (Chapter 9); and (c) effects of friend/family interaction on happiness when persons were isolated/nonisolated from the other type of affiliation (Keith, 1986). To augment earlier analyses and to supply further tests for some of the assumptions discussed above, final assessments of happiness among the formerly married and never married were conducted.

Following suggestions in the literature, these analyses included personal resources and characteristics such as happiness at time 1, education, income, race, health, employment status, interaction with siblings, friends, and participation in formal organizations. Marital status (widowed, divorced) and contact with children were studied among the formerly married. In addition, interaction effects of race and income were investigated for all but never-married men. What conclusions about the happiness of these unmarried then did the various analyses suggest?

In these expanded models, health contributed to the happiness of all of the groups. Regardless of marital status, health was as important or more important than happiness at time 1 in predicting happiness of men later in life. Health figured more prominently in the happiness of men than of women emphasizing again its significance as a massive situational factor that impacts all of life. Although income also is accorded this importance it was less salient for happiness. As observed in Chapter 9, happiness of urban men and women was jeopardized by lower income, for example, but not that of rural people. Giving or receiving financial support from children did not result in either benefits or erosion of happiness, as suggested by some of the theories. By themselves, factors generally thought to indicate social status were not usually the most important in assuring happiness. Separate analyses of happiness by gender and by marital status (formerly married and never married) indicated that higher income directly contributed to contentment expressed only by formerly married women, and then it was not very strong. Income primarily affected happiness through its interaction with race so that widowed and divorced black men and women and never-married black females who fared better economically enjoyed less happiness. Thus economic success constrained and facilitated the happiness of blacks and whites in opposite ways. For these unmarried, higher incomes earned by blacks seemed to be more of a burden than an advantage because the erosion of happiness among blacks who were better off economically was present across all gender and marital status groups for whom it was considered.

There was little evidence that the majority of these unmarried people relied to any great extent on interaction with friends and relatives for their contentment. As shown in Chapter 9, urban women derived some of their happiness from their interaction with friends and siblings, although analyses of each marital status revealed that only the interaction of never-married men with siblings and never-married women with friends contributed somewhat to happiness. Formerly married men and women did not experience increases in happiness when they had contact with children, siblings, or friends. For the most part, then, informal ties had little direct influence on the global happiness expressed by these unmarried. Involvement in formal organizations, such as churches, clubs, and volunteering was reflected in the happiness of only formerly married women, and then it was of secondary importance to other aspects of their lives.

In an extreme instance such as isolation from family, it might be expected that ties with friends would emerge as critical to happiness (Keith, 1986). But relationships with friends were not used to compensate for the absence of family to the degree that they were reflected in happiness. Likewise, interaction with family did not enhance happiness in the absence of friends.

Happiness of those in marital statuses in which loss had occurred was not any more fragile in the face of one kind of loss than another. Following the reasoning of some of the perspectives presented here, women who had lost roles were substantially less happy than women who had not; however, among men the distinction between loss and continuity and their effect on happiness was less marked. As in other areas of life, assessments of happiness reflected the relative advantaged position enjoyed by never-married women.

CONCLUSION

This book has been about men and women who were single for a considerable period of time in their later years, if not for their entire lives. During the most recent years of their singleness, attitudes toward single life seem to have modified somewhat with the occurrence of a general reevaluation of marriage vis-à-vis remaining or becoming unmarried. In the last two decades, persons have become less negative toward being unmarried and see fewer advantages of marriage relative to singleness. Even so, the generally gloomy view of singleness and its presumed negative outcomes were extant throughout most of the lifetime of these older unmarried persons. Clearly though in this rare glimpse of the unmarried over a decade, there was variation across spheres of life in the degree to which marital status was linked to their resources, opportunities, and activities.

Bibliography

Adams, B. *Kinship in an Urban Setting.* Chicago: Markham, 1968.

Adams, M. *Single Blessedness.* New York: Basic Books, 1976.

Alwin, D., Converse, P., and Martin, S. "Living Arrangements and Social Integration." *Journal of Marriage and the Family*, 1985, 47:319-334.

Andersen, R., and Newman, J. "Societal and Individual Determinants of Medical Care Utilization in the United States." *Milbank Memorial Fund Quarterly*, 1973, 51:95-124.

Anderson, T. "Widowhood as a Life Transition; Its Impact on Kinship Ties." *Journal of Marriage and the Family*, 1984, 46:105-114.

Antonucci, T. "Personal Characteristics, Social Support, and Social Behavior." In R. Binstock and E. Shanas (Eds.) *Handbook of Aging and the Social Sciences.* New York: Van Nostrand Reinhold, 1985.

Arens, D. "Widowhood and Well-being: An Examination of Sex Differences within a Causal Model." *International Journal of Aging and Human Development*, 1982-83, 15:27-40.

Arling, G. "The Elderly Widow and Her Family, Neighbors, and Friends." *Journal of Marriage and the Family*, 1976, 38(4):757-768.

Atchley, R. *Social Forces and Aging*, Fifth edition. Belmont, CA: Wadsworth, 1988.

——. *Social Forces and Aging*, Fourth edition. Belmont, CA: Wadsworth, 1985.

——. "The Process of Retirement: Comparing Men and Women." In M. Szinovacz (Ed.) *Women's Retirement: Policy Implications of Recent Research.* Newbury Park, CA: Sage, 1982.

——. "Orientation toward the Job and Retirement Adjustment among Women." In J. Gubrium (Ed.) *Time, Roles, and Self in Old Age.* New York: Human Sciences, 1976.

———. "Selected Social and Psychological Differences between Men and Women in Later Life." *Journal of Gerontology*, 1976, 31:204-212.

———. "Retirement and Work." *The Gerontologist*, 1971, 11, Part 1, 29-32.

Atchley, R., Pignatiello, L., and Shaw, E. C. "Interactions with Family and Friends: Marital Status and Occupational Differences among Older Women." *Research on Aging*, 1979, 1:83-95.

Atchley, R., and Robinson, J. "Attitudes toward Retirement and Distance from the Event." *Research on Aging*, 1982, 4:299-313.

Austrom, D. R. *The Consequences of Being Single*. New York: P. Lang, 1984.

Babchuck, N. "Aging and Primary Relations." *International Journal of Aging and Human Development*, 1978-79, 9:137-151.

Bachrach, C. "Childlessness and Social Isolation among the Elderly." *Journal of Marriage and the Family*, 1980, 42:627-637.

Baldassare, M., Rosenfield, S., and Rook, K. "The Types of Social Relations Predicting Elderly Well-being." *Research on Aging*, 1984, 6(4):549-559.

Ballweg, J. A. "Resolution of Conjugal Role Adjustment After Retirement." *Journal of Marriage and the Family*, 1967, 29:277-281.

Bankoff, E. "Aged Parents and Their Widowed Daughters: A Support Relationship." *Journal of Gerontology*, 1983, 38:226-230.

Barfield, R., and Morgan, J. "Trends in Satisfaction with Retirement." *The Gerontologist*, 1978, 18:19-23.

Beattie, W. "Aging and the Social Services." In R. Binstock and E. Shanas (Eds.) *Handbook of Aging and the Social Sciences*. New York: Van Nostrand Reinhold, 1976.

Beck, S. H. "Adjustment to and Satisfaction with Retirement." *Journal of Gerontology*, 1982, 37:616-624.

Beckman, L., and Houser, B. "The More You Have, The More You Do: The Relationship between Wife's Employment, Sex-role Attitudes, and Household Behavior." *Psychology of Women Quarterly*, 1979, 4:160-174.

Bennett, R. "Introduction, Aging." In R. Bennett (Ed.) *Isolation and Resocialization*. New York: Van Nostrand and Reinhold, 1980.

Berger, P., and Kellner, H. "Marriage and the Construction of Reality." In D. Brissett and C. Edgley (Eds.) *Life as Theatre*. Chicago: Aldine, 1975.

Berheide, C., Berk, F., and Berk, R. "Household Work in the Suburbs." *Pacific Sociological Review*, 1976, 19:491-518.

Berk, R. "Face-Saving at the Singles Dance." *Social Problems*, 1977, 24:530-544.

Bernard, J. *The Future of Marriage*. New York: World, 1972.

Besdine, R. "Health and Illness Behavior in the Elderly." In D. Parron, F. Solomon, and J. Rodin (Eds.) *Health, Behavior, and Aging*. Washington, DC: National Academy Press, 1981.

Birnbaum, J. "Life Patterns and Self-esteem in Gifted Family-oriented and Career-committed Women." In M. Mednick, D. Tangri, and L. Hoffman

(Eds.) *Women and Achievement: Social and Motivational Analyses*. New York: Halsted, 1975.

Blau, Z. *Old Age in a Changing Society*. New York: Franklin Watts, 1973.

Bosse, R., and Ekerdt, D. "Change in Self-Perception of Leisure Activities with Retirement." *The Gerontologist*, 1981, 21:650-654.

Bowling, A., and Cartwright, A. *Life after a Death*. New York: Tavistock, 1982.

Braito, R., and Anderson, D. "The Ever-single Elderly Woman." In E. Markson (Ed.) *Older Women*. Lexington, MA: Lexington, 1983.

———. "Singles and Aging: Implications for Needed Research." In P. Stein (Ed.) *Single Life*. New York: St. Martin's Press, 1981.

Breytspraak, L. M. *The Development of Self in Later Life*. Boston: Little, Brown, 1984.

Brim, O. "Remarks on Life Span Development" presented to the American Institute on Research, 1977. Mimeographed.

Brody, E. "'Women in the Middle' and Family Help to Older People." *The Gerontologist*, 1981, 21:471-480.

Brody, E., Johnsen, P., and Fulcomer, M. "What Should Adult Children do for Elderly Parents? Opinions and Preferences of Three Generations of Women." *Journal of Gerontology*, 1984, 39:736-746.

Brubaker, T. *Later Life Families*. Beverly Hills: Sage, 1985.

——— (Ed.) *Family Relationships in Later Life*. Beverly Hills: Sage, 1983.

Burke, R., and Weir, T. "Relationship of Wives' Employment Status to Husband, Wife and Pair Satisfaction and Performance." *Journal of Marriage and the Family*, 1976, 38:279-287.

Burr, W. "Role Transitions: A Reformulation of Theory." *Journal of Marriage and the Family*, 1972, 24:407-16.

Cafferata, G. "Marital Status, Living Arrangements, and the Use of Health Services by Elderly Persons." *Journal of Gerontology*, 1987, 2:613-618.

———. *Marital Status, Household Structure and the Elderly's Use of Ambulatory Physician Services*. Washington, DC: National Center for Health Services Research, 1984.

Calhoun, A. *A Social History of the American Family*, Vol. 1. Cleveland: Arthur Clark Co., 1917.

Campbell, A. *The Sense of Well-Being in America*. New York: McGraw-Hill, 1981.

Campbell, A., Converse, P., and Rodgers, W. *The Quality of American Life*. New York: Russell Sage, 1976.

Cantor, M., "The Informal Support System: Its Relevance in the Lives of the Elderly." In E. F. Borgatta and N. McCluskey (Eds.) *Aging and Society*. Beverly Hills: Sage, 1980.

Cargan, L., and Melko, M. *Singles: Myths and Realities*. Beverly Hills: Sage, 1982.

Chappell, N. L. "Informal Support Networks among the Elderly." *Research on Aging*, 1983, 5:77-100.

Chappell, N., and Havens, B. "Old and Female: Testing the Double Jeopardy Hypothesis." *The Sociological Quarterly*, 1980, 21:157–171.

Chown, S. "Friendships in Old Age." In S. Duck and R. Gilmour (Eds.) *Personal Relationships*. 2. Developing Personal Relationships. New York: Academic Press, 1981.

Circirelli, V. "Sibling Influence Throughout the Lifespan." In M. Lamb and B. Sutton-Smith (Eds.) *Sibling Relationships: Their Nature and Significance across the Lifespan.* Hillsdale, NJ: Lawrence Erlbaum, 1982.

———. *Helping Elderly Parents*. Boston: Auburn House, 1981.

Clifford, W., Heaton, T., and Fuguitt, G. "Residential Mobility and Living Arrangements among the Elderly: Changing Patterns in Metropolitan and Nonmetropolitan Areas." *International Journal of Aging and Human Development*, 1981–82, 14:139–156.

Cooper, K., and Gutmann, D. "Gender Identity and Ego Mastery Style in Middle-aged, Pre- and Post-empty Nest Women." *The Gerontologist*, 1987, 27: 347–352.

Coulton, C., and Frost, A. "Use of Social and Health Services By the Elderly." *Journal of Health and Social Behavior*, 1982, 23:330–339.

Crawford, M. "Retirement and Disengagement." *Human Relations*, 1971, 24:255–278.

Crosby, F. *Relative Deprivation and Working Women*. New York: Oxford University Press, 1982.

Crossman, L., London, C., and Barry, C. "Older Women Caring for Disabled Spouses: A Model For Supportive Services." *The Gerontologist*, 1981, 21:464–470.

Davis, M., Randall, E., Forthofer, R., Lee, E., and Margen, S. "Living Arrangements and Dietary Patterns of Older Adults in the United States." *Journal of Gerontology*, 1985, 40:434–442.

DeShane, M., and Brown-Wilson, K. "Divorce in Later Life: A Call for Research." *Journal of Divorce*, 1981, 4:81–91.

Donelson, E. "Development of Sex-typed Behavior and Self-concept." In E. Donelson and J. E. Gullahorn (Eds.) *Women*. New York: John Wiley, 1977.

Dowd, J. *Stratification among the Aged*. Monterey, CA: Brooks-Cole, 1980.

Duberman, L. *Marriage and Other Alternatives*. New York: Praeger, 1977.

Edwards, J., and Klemmack, D. "Correlates of Life Satisfaction: A Re-examination." *Journal of Gerontology*, 1973, 28:497–502.

Elwell, F., and Maltbie-Crannell, A. "The Impact of Role Loss upon Coping Resources and Life Satisfaction of the Elderly." *Journal of Gerontology*, 1981, 36:223–232.

Etaugh, C., and Malstrom, J. "The Effect of Marital Status on Person Perception." *Journal of Marriage and the Family*, 1981, 43:801–805.

Fengler, A., Danigelis, N., and Little, V. "Later Life Satisfaction and Household Structure: Living with Others and Living Alone." *Aging and Society*, 1983, 3(3):357–377.

Fenwick, R., and Barresi, C. "Health Consequences of Marital-status Change Among the Elderly: A Comparison of Cross-sectional and Longitudinal Analyses." *Journal of Health and Social Behavior*, 1981, 22:106-116.

Fillenbaum, G. "On the Relation between Attitude to Work and Attitude to Retirement." *Journal of Gerontology*, 1971, 26:244-248.

Fillenbaum, G., and Wallman, L. "Change in Household Composition of the Elderly: A Preliminary Investigation." *Journal of Gerontology*, 1984, 39:342-349.

Finch, J., and Groves, D. *A Labour of Love*. London: Routledge and Kegan Paul, 1983.

Fischer, C. *To Dwell among Friends*. Chicago: University of Chicago Press, 1982.

Fischer, C., and Phillips, S. "Who is Alone? Social Characteristics of People with Small Networks." In L. Peplau and D. Perlman (Eds.) *Loneliness: A Sourcebook of Current Theory, Research, and Therapy*. New York: Wiley, 1982.

Foner, A. *Aging and Old Age*. Englewood Cliffs, NJ: Prentice-Hall, 1986.

Foner, A., and Schwab, K. *Aging and Retirement*. Monterey, CA: Brooks/Cole, 1981.

Fox, J. "Effects of Retirement and Former Work on Women's Adaptation in Old Age." *Journal of Gerontology*, 1977, 32:196-202.

Frank, S. J., Towell, P. A., and Huyck, M. "The Effects of Sex-role Traits on Three Aspects of Psychological Well-being in a Sample of Middle-aged Women." *Sex Roles*, 1985, 12:1073-1087.

Franklin, B. "Advice to a Young Man on Choosing a Mistress." 1745. In L. Labare and W. Bell, Jr. (Eds.) *The Papers of Benjamin Franklin*, Vol. 3. New Haven, CT: Yale University Press, 1961.

Friedman, J., and Sjogren, J. "The Assets of the Elderly as They Retire." *Social Security Bulletin*, 1981, 44:16-31.

Gallup Report. "What's Important to Americans." Report, March, 1982.

Gee, E., and Kimball, M. *Women and Aging*. Toronto: Butterworths, 1987.

Gilder, G. *Naked Nomads*. New York: Quadrangle, 1974.

Glamser, F. "Determinants of a Positive Attitude toward Retirement." *Journal of Gerontology*, 1976, 31:104-107.

Glenn, N. "The Contribution of Marriage to the Psychological Well-being of Males and Females." *Journal of Marriage and the Family*, 1975, 37:594-601.

Glenn, N., and McLanahan, S. "Children and Marital Happiness: A Further Specification of the Relationship." *Journal of Marriage and the Family*, 1982, 44:217-224.

———. "The Effects of Offspring on the Psychological Well-Being of Older Adults." *Journal of Marriage and the Family*, 1981, 43:409-421.

Glick, P. "The Future Marital Status and Living Arrangements of the Elderly." *The Gerontologist*, 1979, 19(3):301-309.

Goudy, W., Powers, E., and Keith, P. "Work and Retirement: A Test of Attitudinal Relationships." *Journal of Gerontology*, 1975, 30:193-198.

Gratton, B., and Haug, M. "Decision and Adaptation: Research on Female Retirement." *Research on Aging*, 1983, 5:59-76.

Gubrium, J. "Being Single in Old Age." *International Journal of Aging and Human Development*, 1975, 6:29-40.

Gutmann, D. "Parenthood: A Key to the Comparative Study of the Life Cycle." In N. Datan and L. H. Ginsberg (Eds.) *Life-Span Developmental Psychology*. New York: Academic Press, 1975.

Gutmann, D. L. "Psychoanalysis and Aging: A Developmental View." In S. I. Greenspan and G. H. Pollack (Eds.) *The Cause of Life: Psychoanalytic Contributions toward Understanding Personality Development*, Vol. 3. Washington, DC: National Institute of Mental Health, 1980.

Haberman, S. *Analysis of Qualitative Data*, Vol. 1. New York: Academic Press, 1978.

Harris, L., and Associates. *Aging in the Eighties: America in Transition*. Washington, DC: National Council on the Aging, 1981.

Hatch, L. "Research on Men's and Women's Retirement Attitudes." In E. Borgotta and R. Montgomery (Eds.) *Critical Issues in Aging Policy*. Newbury Park, CA: Sage, 1987.

Haug, M. "Age and Medical Care Utilization Patterns." *Journal of Gerontology*, 1981, 33:103-111.

Havens, E. M. "Women, Work and Wedlock: A Note on Female Marital Patterns in the United States." *American Journal of Sociology*, 1973, 78(4):975-981.

Havighurst, R. *Developmental Tasks and Education*. New York: McKay, 1972.

Hennon, C. "Divorce and the Elderly: A Neglected Area of Research." In T. Brubaker (Ed.) *Family Relationships in Later Life.* Beverly Hills: Sage, 1983.

Hess, B. "America's Elderly: A Demographic Overview." In B. Hess and E. Markson (Eds.) *Growing Old in America, New Perspectives on Old Age*. New Brunswick, NJ: Rutgers, 1985.

Hess, B., and Waring, J. "Family Relations of Older Women: A Women's Issue." In E. Markson (Ed.) *Older Women*. Lexington, MA: Lexington, 1983.

Hickey, I. *Health and Aging*. Monterey, CA: Brooks/Cole, 1980.

Holzer, C., Leaf, P., and Weissman, M. "Living With Depression." In M. Haug, A. Ford, and M. Sheafor (Eds.) *The Physical and Mental Health of Aged Women*. New York: Springer, 1985.

House, J. "Social Support." *Institute for Social Research Newsletter*, Autumn 1984, University of Michigan.

House, J., and Robbins, C. "Age, Psychosocial Stress, and Health." In M. Riley, B. Hess, and K. Bond (Eds.) *Aging in Society: Selected Reviews of Recent Research*. Hillsdale, NJ: Lawrence Erlbaum Associates, 1983.

Hughes, M., and Gove, W. "Living Alone, Social Contact and Psychological Well-being." *American Journal of Society*, 1981, 87:48-74.

Hyman, H. *Of Time and Widowhood*. Durham, NC: Duke Press Policy Studies, 1983.

Iijima, Y. *Incidence of Poverty among Elderly Men and Women*. Doctoral Dissertation, Iowa State University, 1987.

Irelan, L. "Retirement History Study: Introduction." *Social Security Bulletin*, 1972, 35:3-9.

Janigian, A., Paloutzian, R., and Thompson, S. "Is Loneliness a Discrepancy between What One Wants and What One Gets?" Presented at the Second National Conference on Stress, University of New Hampshire, 1986.

Jaslow, P. "Employment, Retirement, and Morale among Older Women." *Journal of Gerontology*, 1976, 31:212-218.

Johnson, C. "Dyadic Family Relations and Social Support." *The Gerontologist*, 1983, 23:377-383.

Johnson, C., and Catalano, D. "Childless Elderly and Their Family Supports." *The Gerontologist*, 1981, 21:610-618.

Johnson, E., and Williamson, J. "Retirement in the United States." In K. Markides and C. Cooper (Eds.) *Retirement in Industrialized Societies*. Chichester: John Wiley and Sons, 1987.

Keating, N., and Jeffrey, B. "Work Careers of Ever-married and Never-married Retired Women." *The Gerontologist*, 1983, 23:416-421.

Keith, P. "Isolation of the Unmarried in Later Life." *Family Relations*, 1986, 35:389-397.

———. "The Social Context and Resources of the Unmarried in Old Age." *International Journal of Aging and Human Development*, 1986, 23:81-96.

———. "Change in Life Areas and Well-being." In E. Powers, W. Goudy, and P. Keith (Eds.) *Older Workers in Small Towns*. Boston: Kluwer-Nijhoff, 1985.

———. "Importance of Life Areas." In E. Powers, W. Goudy, and P. Keith (Eds.) *Later Life Transitions*. Boston: Kluwer-Nijhoff, 1985.

Keith, P., and Lorenz, F. "Financial Strain and Health among the Unmarried Aged." Presented at the Midwest Sociological Society, 1985.

Keith, P., Powers, E., and Goudy, W. "Older Men in Employed and Retired Families." *Alternative Lifestyles*, 1981, 4:228-241.

Keith, P., and Schafer, R. "Housework, Disagreement, and Depression among Younger and Older Couples." *American Behavioral Scientist*, 1986, 29:405-422.

Keith, P., and Wacker, R. "Gender Roles in the Elderly Family: Implications for Mental Health." Presented at the Midwest Sociological Society, 1988.

Kelly, J. R., Steinkamp, M., and Kelly, J. "Later Life Leisure—How They Play in Peoria." *Gerontologist*, 1986, 26(5):531-537.

Kimmel, D. *Adulthood and Aging*. New York: John Wiley, 1974.

Kitson, G., Lopata, H., Holmes, W., and Meyerling, S. "Divorcees and Widows: Similarities and Differences." *American Journal of Orthopsychiatry*, 1980, 50:291–301.

Kivett, V. "Aging in Rural Society: Non-kin Community Relations and Participation." In R. Coward and G. Lee (Eds.) *The Elderly in Rural Society*. New York: Springer, 1985.

Kohen, J. "Old But Not Alone: Informal Social Supports among the Elderly by Marital Status and Sex." *Gerontologist*, 1983, 23:57-63.

Kremer, Y., and Harpaz, I. "Leisure Patterns among Retired Workers: Spillover or Compensatory Trends." *Journal of Vocational Behavior*, 1982, 21:183–195.

Krout, J. *The Aged in Rural America*. Westport, CT: Greenwood, 1986.

Kuhn, M. "How Mates are Sorted." In H. Becker and R. Hill (Eds.) *Family, Marriage, and Parenthood*. Boston: D. C. Heath, 1948.

Larson, R. "Thirty Years of Research on the Subjective Well-being of Older Americans." *Journal of Gerontology*, 1978, 33:109–125.

Lawton, M. "An Ecological View of Living Arrangements." *The Gerontologist*, 1981, 21(1):59-66.

Lawton, M., Moss, M., and Kleban, M. "Marital Status, Living Arrangements, and the Well-being of Older People." *Research on Aging*, 1984, 6(3):323-345.

Lee, G. "Kinship and Social Support of the Elderly: The Case of the United States." *Aging and Society*, 1985, 5:19-38.

Lee, G., and Cassidy, M. "Family and Kin Relations of the Rural Elderly." In R. Coward and G. Lee (Eds.) *The Elderly in Rural Society*. New York: Springer, 1985.

Lee, G., and Ellithorpe, E. "Intergenerational Exchange and Subjective Well-being among the Elderly." *Journal of Marriage and the Family*, 1982, 46:217-224.

Lee, G., and Lassley, M. "The Elderly." In D. Dillman and D. Hobbs (Eds.) *Rural Society in the U.S.: Issues For the 1980s*. Boulder, CO: Westview Press, 1982.

Lee, G., and Whitbeck, L. "Residential Location and Social Relations among Older Persons." *Rural Sociology*, 1987, 52:89-97.

Levy, S. "The Adjustment of the Older Woman: Effects of Chronic Ill Health and Attitudes toward Retirement." *International Journal of Aging and Human Development*, 1980, 12:93-110.

Liang, J., Kahana, E., and Doherty, E. "Financial Well-being among the Aged: A Further Elaboration." *Journal of Gerontology*, 1980, 35:409-420.

Liang, J., and Warfel, B. "Urbanism and Life Satisfaction among the Aged." *Journal of Gerontology*, 1983, 38:97-106.

Lieberman, M. "Social Psychological Determinants of Adaptation." *International Journal of Aging and Human Development*, 1978-79, 9(2):115-126.

Lipman, A. "Role Conceptions and Morale of Couples in Retirement." *Journal of Gerontology*, 1961, 16:267-271.

Livson, F. B. "Changing Sex Roles in the Social Environment of Later Life." In G. D. Rowles and R. J. Ohta (Eds.) *Aging and Milieu: Environmental Perspectives in Growing Old*. New York: Academic Press, 1983.

Longino, C., and Lipman, A. "Married and Spouseless Men and Women in Planned Retirement Communities: Support Network Differentials." *Journal of Marriage and the Family*, 1981, 43:169-177.

Lowenthal, M., Thurner, M., and Chiriboga, D. *Four Stages of Life*. San Francisco: Jossey-Bass, 1975.

Maddox, G., and Douglass, E. "Aging and Individual Differences: A Longitudinal Analysis of Social Psychological and Physiological Indicators." *Journal of Gerontology*, 1974, 44:3-11.

Marsh, R. "The Income and Resources of the Elderly in 1978." *Social Security Bulletin*, 1981, 44:3-31.

Matthews, A., and Brown, K. "Retirement as a Critical Life Event." *Research on Aging*, 1987, 9:548-571.

McBroom, W. "Longitudinal Change in Sex Role Orientations: Differences between Men and Women." *Sex Roles*, 1987, 16:439-452.

McKinlay, J. "Social Network Influences on Morbid Episodes and the Career of Help Seeking." In L. Eisenberg and A. Kleinman (Eds.) *The Relevance of Social Science for Medicine*. Dordrecht, Holland: D. Reidel Co., 1981.

McPherson, B. D. *Aging as a Social Process: An Introduction to Individual and Population Aging*. Toronto: Butterworths, 1983.

Mechanic, D. "Correlates of Physician Utilization: Why Do Major Multivariate Studies of Physician Utilization Find Trivial Psychological and Organizational Effects?" *Journal of Health and Social Behavior*, 1979, 20:387-396.

Mindel, C. "Multigenerational Family Households: Recent Trends and Implications for the Future." *The Gerontologist*, 1979, 19(5):456-463.

Mindel, C., and Wright, R. "Satisfaction in Multigenerational Households." *Journal of Gerontology*, 1982a, 37(4):483-489.

———. "Differential Living Arrangements among the Elderly and Their Subjective Well-being." *Activities, Adaptation, and Aging*, 1982b, 3(2):25-34.

Minnigerode, F., and Lee, J. "Young Adults' Perceptions of Social Sex Roles across the Life Span." *Sex Roles*, 1978, 4:563-569.

Moore, F. "New Issues For In-home Services." *Public Welfare*, 1977, 35:26-27.

Morgan, L. "Economic Change at Mid-life Widowhood: A Longitudinal Analysis." *Journal of Marriage and the Family*, 1981, 43:899-907.

Morgan, C. S., Affleck, M., and Riggs, L. R. "Gender, Personality Traits and Depression." *Social Science Quarterly*, 1986, 67:69-81.

Morris, J., and Sherwood, S. "Informal Support Resources for Vulnerable Elderly Persons: Can They Be Counted on, Why Do They Work?" *International Journal of Aging and Human Development*, 1983-84, 18:81-98.

Mouser, N. F., Powers, E. A., Keith, P. M., and Goudy, W. J. "Marital Status and Life Satisfaction: A Study of Older Men." In W. A. Peterson and J. Quadagno (Eds.) *Social Bonds in Later Life*. Beverly Hills: Sage, 1985.

Mutran, E., and Reitzes, D. C. "Retirement, Identity and Well-being: Realignment of Role Relationships." *Journal of Psychology*, 1981, 36:733-740.

Nash, S. C., and Feldman, S. S. "Sex Role and Sex Related Attributions: Constancy and Change Across the Family Life Cycle." In M. E. Lamb and A. L. Brown (Eds.) *Advances in Developmental Psychology*, Vol. 1. Hillsdale, NJ: Lea, 1981.

National Center for Health Statistics, U.S. Dept. HEW, United States. DHEW Pub. No. (PHS)78-1232. Hyattsville, MD: Public Health Service, 1978.

Nimkoff, M. F. *The Family*. New York: Houghton Mifflin, 1934.

Norton, A. "Keeping up with Households." *American Demographics*, 1983, 17-21.

Norton, A., and Moorman, J. "Current Trends in Marriage and Divorce among American Women." *Journal of Marriage and the Family*, 1987, 49:3-14.

Nyguist, L., Slivken, K., Sperse, J. T., and Helmreich, R. L. "Household Responsibilities in Middle-class Couples: The Contribution of Demographic and Personality Variables." *Sex Roles*, 1985, 12:15-34.

Oakley, A. *The Sociology of Housework*. London: The Pitman Press, 1974.

O'Bryant, S. "Neighbors' Support of Older Widows Who Live Alone in Their Own Homes." *The Gerontologist*, 1985, 25(3):305-310.

O'Rand, A. "Women." In E. Palmore (Ed.) *Handbook on the Aged in the United States*. Westport, CT: Greenwood, 1984.

Palmore, E. *Social Patterns in Normal Aging: Findings from the Duke Longitudinal Study*. Durham: Duke University Press, 1981.

———. "Total Chance of Institutionalization among the Aged." *The Gerontologist*, 1976, 16:504-507.

Palmore, E. B., Fillenbaum, G. G., and George, K. L. "Consequences of Retirement." *Journal of Gerontology*, 1984, 39:109-116.

Pearlin, L., and Johnson, J. "Marital Status, Life Strains and Depression." *American Sociological Review*, 1977, 42:704-715.

Perlman, D., and Peplau, L. "Loneliness Research: A Survey of Empirical Findings." In L. Peplau and D. Perlman (Eds.) *Preventing the Harmful Consequences of Severe and Persistent Loneliness*. Rockville, MD: U.S. Department of Health and Human Services, 1984.

Peters, J., and Haldeman, V. "Time Used for Household Work." *Journal of Family Issues*, 1987, 8:212-225.

Pleck, J. "Husbands' Paid Work and Family Roles: Current Research Issues." In H. Lopata and J. Pleck (Eds.) *Research in the Interweave of Social Roles: Jobs and Families*, 3:251-333. Greenwich: JAI Press, 1983.

Puglisi, T. "Self-Perceived Age Changes in Sex Role Self Concept." *International Journal of Aging and Human Development*, 1983, 16:183-191.

Rapoport, R., and Rapoport, R. *Leisure and the Life Cycle*. London: Routledge and Kegan Paul, 1975.

Riddick, C. "Life Satisfaction among Aging Women: The Experience of the

Mature Woman." In M. Szinovacz (Ed.) *Women's Retirement*. Beverly Hills: Sage Publications, 1982.

——. "Life Satisfaction for Older Female Homemakers, Retirees, and Workers." *Research on Aging*, 1985, 3:383-393.

Roadburg, A. "Perceptions of Work and Leisure among the Elderly." *The Gerontologist*, 1981, 21:142-145.

Roberto, K., and J. Scott. "Confronting Widowhood." *American Behavioral Scientist*, 1986, 29:497-511.

Robinson, J. *How Americans Use Time*. New York: Praeger, 1977.

Rook, K. "Promoting Social Bonding." *American Psychologist*, 1984, 39:1389-1407.

Rubinstein, R. *Singular Paths: Old Men Living Alone*. New York: Columbia University Press, 1986.

Rubinstein, R. "The Elderly Who Live Alone and Their Social Supports." In M. P. Lawton and G. Maddox (Eds.) *Annual Review of Gerontology and Geriatrics*. New York: Springer, 1985.

Ruhlenberg, P., and Myers, M. "Divorce and the Elderly." *The Gerontologist*, 1981, 21:276-282.

Schafer, R., Keith, P., and Lorenz, F. "A Causal Model Approach to the Symbolic Interactionist View of the Self-Concept." *Journal of Personality and Social Psychology*, 1984, 48:963-969.

Schnore, M. *Retirement: Bane or Blessing?* Waterloo, Ontario: Wilfrid Laurier University Press, 1985.

Seccombe, K., and Lee, G. R. "Gender Differences in Retirement Satisfaction and Its Antecedents." *Research on Aging*, 1986, 8:426-440.

Seelbach, W. "Correlates of Aged Parents' Filial Responsibility Expectations and Realizations." *The Family Coordinator*, 1978, 27:341-350.

Seelbach, W., and Sauer, W. "Filial Responsibility Expectations and Morale among Aged Parents." *The Gerontologist*, 1977, 17:492-499.

Seltzer, M. "Suggestions for the Examination of Time-disordered Relationships." In J. Gubrium (Ed.) *Time, Roles, and Self in Old Age*. New York: Human Sciences Press, 1976.

Shanas, E. "Older People and Their Families: The New Pioneers." *Journal of Marriage and the Family*, 1980, 42:9-15.

——. "The Family as a Social Support System in Old Age." *The Gerontologist*, 1979, 19:169-174.

Shanas, E., and Maddox, G. "Aging, Health, and the Organization of Health Resources." In R. Binstock and E. Shanas (Eds.) *Handbook of Aging and the Social Sciences*. New York: Van Nostrand Reinhold, 1976.

Shuval, J. *The Social Functions of Medical Practice*. San Francisco, CA: Jossey-Bass, 1970.

Sinnott, J. D. *Sex Roles and Aging: Theory and Research from a Systems Perspective*. Basel, New York: Kargen, 1986.

————. "Sex-role Inconsistency, Biology, and Successful Aging." *The Gerontologist*, 1977, 5(17):459–463.

Sivley, J., and Fiegener, J. "Family Caregivers of the Elderly: Assistance Provided after Termination of Chore Services." *Journal of Gerontological Social Work*, 1984, 8:23–24.

Soldo, B., Mahesh, S., and Campbell, R. "Determinants of the Community Living Arrangements of Older Unmarried Women." *Journal of Gerontology*, 1984, 39(4):492–498.

Spence, J., Deaux, K., and Helmreich, R. "Sex Roles in Contemporary American Society." In G. Lindzey and E. Aronson (Eds.) *Handbook of Social Psychology*, Vol. 3. New York: Random House, 1985.

Spreitzer, E., and Riley, L. "Factors Associated with Singlehood." *Journal of Marriage and the Family*, 1974, 36:533–542.

Stafford, R., Backman, E., and DiBona, P. "The Division of Labor among Cohabitating and Married Couples." *Journal of Marriage and the Family*, 1977, 39:43–57.

Stein, P. "Understanding Single Adulthood." In P. Stein (Ed.) *Single Life*. New York: St. Martin's Press, 1981.

————. "The Lifestyles and Life Chances of the Never-married." *Marriage and Family Review*, 1978, 1:2–11.

————. *Single*. Englewood Cliffs, NJ: Prentice-Hall, 1976.

Stoller, S. "Parental Caregiving By Adult Children." *Journal of Marriage and the Family*, 1983, 45:851–858.

Streib, G. "The Frail Elderly: Research Dilemmas and Research Opportunities." *The Gerontologist*, 1983, 23:40–44.

Streib, G., and Schneider, C. *Retirement in American Society Impact and Process*. Ithaca, NY: Cornell University Press, 1971.

Stroebe, M., and Stroebe, W. "Who Suffers More? Sex Differences in Health Risks of the Widowed." *Psychological Bulletin*, 1983, 93:179–301.

Szinovacz, M. "Beyond the Hearth: Older Women and Retirement." In E. Markson (Ed.) *Older Women*. Lexington, MA: Lexington, 1983.

————. "Introduction: Research on women's retirement." In M. Szinovacz (Ed.) *Women's Retirement: Policy Implications of Recent Research*. Beverly Hills: Sage, 1982.

Tessler, R., Mechanic, D., and Dimond, J. "The Effect of Psychological Distress on Physician Utilization: A Prospective Study." *Journal of Health and Social Behavior*, 1976, 17:353–364.

Thomas, K., and Wister, A. "Living Arrangements of Older Women: The Ethnic Dimension." *Journal of Marriage and the Family*, 1984, 46(2):301–311.

Thornton, A., and Freedman, D. *The Changing American Family*. Population Reference Bureau, Vol. 38, No. 4, October, 1983.

Tissue, T., and McCoy, J. "Income Living Arrangements among Poor Singles." *Social Security Bulletin*, 1981, 44:3–13.

Uhlenberg, P., and Myers, M. "Divorce and the Elderly." *The Gerontologist*, 1981, 21:276–282.

U.S. Bureau of the Census. "Marital Status and Living Arrangements: March, 1985." *Current Population Reports*, Series P-20, No. 410 (Nov). Washington, DC: Government Printing Office, 1986.

——. *Statistical Abstract of the United States*, 1981. Washington, DC: Government Printing Office, 1981.

——. *Statistical Abstract of the United States*. Washington, DC: Government Printing Office, 1979, 1986.

——. *Historical Statistics of the United States, Colonial Times to 1970*. Washington, DC: Government Printing Office, 1975.

U.S. Department of Commerce. "Marital Status and Living Arrangements: March, 1982." In U.S. Bureau of the Census *Current Population Reports*, Series P-20, No. 380. Washington, DC: Government Printing Office, 1983.

Veenhoven, R. *Conditions of Happiness*. Dordrecht, Holland: D. Reidel Co., 1984.

Veevers, J. "The Moral Careers of Voluntarily Childless Wives: Notes on the Defense of a Variant World View." *The Family Coordinator*, 1975, 24: 473–487.

Verbrugge, L. "Gender and Health: An Update on Hypotheses and Evidence." *Journal of Health and Social Behavior*, 1985, 26:156–182.

——. "A Health Profile of Older Women with Comparisons to Older Men." *Research on Aging*, 1984, 6(3):291–322.

——. "Marital Status and Health." *Journal of Marriage and the Family*, 1979, 41:267–285.

Veroff, J., Douvan, E., and Kulka, C. *The Inner American*. New York: Basic Books, 1981.

Wakil, S. P. "To Be or Not To Be Married." *International Journal of Sociology of the Family*, 1980, 10:311–318.

Walker, J., Kimmel, D., and Price, K. "Retirement Style and Retirement Satisfaction: Retirees Aren't All Alike." *International Journal of Aging and Human Development*, 1980–81, 12:267–281.

Wan, T. *Stressful Life Events, Social-Support Networks, and Gerontological Health*. Lexington, MA: Lexington Books, 1982.

Ward, R. *The Aging Experience*. New York: Harper and Row, 1984.

——. "The Never-married in Later Life." *Journal of Gerontology*, 1979, 34: 861–869.

——. "Services for Older People: An Integrated Framework for Research." *Journal of Health and Social Behavior*, 1977, 18:61–70.

Warlick, J. "Why Is Poverty after 65 a Woman's Problem?" *Journal of Gerontology*, 1985, 40:751–757.

Wenger, C. "Adapting to Old Age in Rural Britain." *International Journal of Aging and Human Development*, 1981, 19:287–299.

Whicker, M., and Kronenfeld, J. *Sex Role Changes*. New York: Praeger, 1986.

Williamson, J. B., Evans, L., and Munley, A., in collaboration with Vinick, B. H., and Hesse, S. *Aging and Society*. New York: Holt, Rinehart and Winston, 1980.

Willmott, P., and Young, M. *Family and Class in a London Suburb*. London: Routledge and Kegan Paul, 1960.

Windle, M. "Sex Role Orientation, Cognitive Flexibility, and Life Satisfaction Among Older Adults." *Psychology of Women Quarterly*, 1986, 10:263-273.

Wolinsky, F., and Coe, R. "Physician and Hospital Utilization among Noninstitutionalized Elderly Adults: An Analysis of the Health Interview Survey." *Journal of Gerontology*, 1984, 39:334-341.

Wood, V., and Sheafor, B. "An Analysis of a Short Report Measure of Life Satisfaction: Correlation with Later Judgments." *Journal of Gerontology*, 1969, 24:465-469.

Zick, C., and Smith, K. "Immediate and Delayed Effects of Widowhood on Poverty: Patterns from the 1970s." *The Gerontologist*, 1986, 26:669-675.

Index